Muscular Retraining for Pain-Free Living

Muscular Retraining
for Pain-Free Living

Craig Williamson, MSOT

Trumpeter
Boston & London
2007

Trumpeter Books
An imprint of Shambhala Publications, Inc.
Horticultural Hall
300 Massachusetts Avenue
Boston, Massachusetts 02115
www.shambhala.com

The information in this book is not intended as a substitute for
personalized medical advice. The reader should consult a physician
before beginning this or any exercise program. If you experience
increased pain during or after these exercises, it may indicate a
problem that requires the attention of your physician.

9 8 7 6 5 4 3

Printed in the United States of America

♾ This edition is printed on acid-free paper that meets the American
National Standards Institute z39.48 Standard.

Distributed in the United States by Random House, Inc., and in
Canada by Random House of Canada Ltd

Interior design and composition: Greta D. Sibley & Associates

Library of Congress Cataloging-in-Publication Data
Williamson, Craig.
Muscular retraining for pain-free living/Craig Williamson—1st ed.
p.   cm.
Includes index.
ISBN 978-1-59030-367-2 (pbk.)
1. Myalgia—Treatment—Popular works. 2. Exercise therapy—
Popular works. I. Title.
RC925.5.W55 2007
616.7'4206—DC22
2006053283

Dedicated to Maria Schnaitman

Contents

Introduction

FIFTY-FIVE-YEAR-OLD KEVIN came to my office after hearing about me from a friend. Kevin's doctor had recently told him that the lower back pain he had been feeling for months was caused by a combination of bulging and compressed discs in his lumbar spine. When I first saw him, he was a bit hunched over, walking with the typical protective posture of someone trying to avoid a sharp pain with every step.

Kevin had been an athlete his entire life. In recent years, he had been playing a lot of tennis and running four times a week. The pain in his lower back came on gradually over the course of several months. When I met him, he was spending most of his time lying down, and tennis and running were out of the question.

I taught Kevin how to relax his back muscles, how to use his abdominal muscles, and how to improve the alignment of his back and hips. I did this by first teaching him how to feel his muscles and to become aware of what they were actually doing. Despite being an athlete, Kevin—like most of the people who come to my office—was out of touch with his body. That changed quickly as a result of the exercises I taught him, all of which are included in this book.

Kevin learned how to sit and stand without overcompressing his lower back. Not rocket science, but since he had never learned about it before, it turned out to be of immeasurable importance to him. Within a month of beginning the exercises, he reported that the low back pain was no longer constant. After two months, he said that the pain occurred only intermittently or when he twisted too far in one direction. After four months, he told me that the pain was pretty much gone. After six months, he began running again. Ten years later, Kevin is still running and has no back pain.

Does this sound like fantasy or reality?

Physical movement is inherently pleasurable, yet many people do not experience it that way. If you spend some time at a playground with preschool children, you can't help but notice that most of them enjoy running, jumping, and moving in all kinds of ways. For adults, the main issue that interferes with the enjoyment of movement is physical pain.

To enjoy working in your garden, painting your house, carrying your child, or driving your car, you need to be able to move without pain. Some people seem to manage for a while by taking painkillers. But drugs simply mask the symptoms without addressing the cause of the pain. Unless the cause is addressed, symptoms tend to worsen over time. Ultimately, the experience, fear, and anticipation of pain inhibit an individual's activity. This means doing less work around the house, playing less frequently with children or grandchildren, getting less exercise, and so on. I tell people who suffer from chronic or recurring pain that their body is not an enemy. I show them what they need to know in order to make their body an ally. I tell them—and I am telling you now—that it is possible to change.

When you are free from physical pain, you are able to enjoy the simple pleasures of movement—from gardening to basketball and everything in between. When you are able to use your body without pain, you enjoy a sense of well-being.

From early in my childhood, I can remember always enjoying giving and receiving back massages. When I was twenty years old, I had my first massage from a trained massage therapist. This was a profound experience of relaxation that began a lifelong pursuit to understand how to achieve well-being, for both myself and others.

I first studied massage therapy in Boston in 1979 and moved to Nantucket Island shortly thereafter. One year later, I had a private practice there. I was in the right place at the right time, because the public was just beginning to get an inkling of the health value of massage treatments. I focused on general relaxation massage therapy, but I also had many clients who were dealing with recurring pain, such as lower backache and stiff shoulders. These clients would leave my office happily rid of their aches and pains, but they would return regularly because of the same problems. From a business point of view, these repeat customers were a virtual guarantee that I would never be without work. Nevertheless, I soon became dissatisfied with my inability to offer a more permanent solution to my clients' muscular pain. I began to inquire into the cause of common bodily discomfort. This turned out to be an enormous question, which led to an ongoing study of bodywork techniques that addressed difficult musculoskeletal problems more effectively than the basic massage skills I already knew.

For the next five years, I traveled back and forth across the country, attending seminars and lengthy training programs where I learned a great deal about body therapies. Many of the techniques I learned, such as connective tissue manipulation and acupressure, were relatively unknown back then but have since become widely used. I investigated every method that made any sense to me. I became quite good with my hands, and I could work effectively with difficult problems that massage therapy alone could not address.

My training continued through the 1980s. During this time, I realized that movement and psychology had as much to do with bodily pain as muscle trigger points. It was then that I began exploring how to use yoga and tai chi exercises to increase both physical health and body awareness. I also completed a psychotherapy course, which greatly expanded my understanding of bodywork.

As a result of all this training, I realized that there was a common thread between body movement, self-awareness, and relaxation. I began to recognize that most of my clients lacked the specific ability to sense their own movement accurately. This sense of movement is known as the *kinesthetic sense,* or kinesthetic awareness. I made a startling discovery: if I could help a client increase kinesthetic awareness, entire muscle groups that had been tense for years would sometimes release within minutes. I began using kinesthetic awareness to investigate my own long-standing back problems that had resulted from numerous injuries. I was my own laboratory.

Toward the end of the 1980s, the many influences of the previous ten years began to fall into place. I began to develop new corrective exercises, educational techniques, and hands-on techniques that pulled together everything I had learned, integrating many different theories of therapy and exercise. I spent hundreds of hours moving slowly on the floor, working out different exercises. If a therapeutic technique worked for me, I would introduce it to my clients to see if it produced a reliable result. Following this simple process of discovery-and-trial, my method evolved. Without intentional planning, I had discovered a new way of working with individual clients and students in group classes, using a combination of hands-on techniques, movement awareness exercises, and alignment education. A great side benefit to this was that I solved my own problem of recurring severe lower back pain all by myself. The resounding success in ending my own pain made me living proof that kinesthetic awareness could be used to make physical changes.

I have maintained an independent practice in Portland, Maine, since 1986. Although the methods I use have helped thousands of people with pain, many of them for months or years, they are not intended to reverse genuine structural injuries—those that call for surgery or other forms of conventional medical treatment. My approach is extremely effective in treating musculoskeletal problems that stem from habitual muscle strain, high-impact accidents, rigid posture, athletic injury, repetitive motion, and psychological stress. Many of my clients are referred to me by medical doctors when conventional approaches have failed to fully alleviate their pain.

Frequently, I demonstrate a simple technique that immediately and dramatically reduces a person's pain and stiffness. However, it sometimes takes months of home exercises and bodywork to solve the problem.

When I work with an individual, I use a combination of movement exercises, education, and hands-on manipulation. The hands-on techniques are very specialized and therefore are not the focus of this book. Fortunately, many people need little or no hands-on treatment to realize the benefits of these exercises. Most readers will be able to use a combination of conceptual understanding and experiential learning to make actual changes to their musculoskeletal system. On the conceptual side is an intellectual understanding of how the body, mind, and psyche interact to create both movement and pain. Experiential learning, on the other hand, is the result of consciously doing the neuromuscular retraining exercises.

Time and again, people tell me, "If I had learned this when I was younger, it would have saved me a lot of trouble," or "I didn't know that this was possible. Why haven't I heard about this before?" Clients often ask, "Is there a book about this that I can read?" After years of hearing these questions, I decided to write this book. My wish is to make this profoundly practical information about muscles, movement, and the mind-body connection available to anyone and everyone who might benefit from it.

Another goal of this book is to demystify the problems of dealing with muscular pain, so that you can understand the cause of your pain and take an active role in achieving well-being. My goal for you, the reader, is the same as for my clients and students: to help you become as autonomous as possible. The better you understand and feel the purpose of the different exercises, the more able you will be to solve your pain problem. As a result, you will be able to increase your enjoyment of movement, reduce the pain and inflexibility that interfere with your ability to move naturally, and improve your emotional well-being by increasing your awareness.

This book contains the concepts and exercises I have learned, discovered, and developed in more than twenty years of working with people who have muscular pain. My hope is for you to learn about the connection between your nervous system (mind) and your muscular system (body) and to use this understanding to become aware of how you may have developed dysfunctional muscle habits that now cause you tension and pain.

The information in this book provides a foundation on which you can establish a beneficial approach to exercise and physical fitness. My clients often ask me how they would benefit from a particular kind of exercise—yoga, weight training, tai chi, swimming, aerobics, running, martial arts, walking, and so forth. All forms of exercise can be useful and even life-changing if approached with awareness. To know what kind of exercise might work best for you in your particular circumstances, you first need to understand how your body works. What are muscle tension, strength, and relaxation, and how are they important? What is the basis of good body alignment? Why do you develop the habit of tense or slouchy posture? Why are you prone to muscle strain? Why don't you feel right after recovering from a minor injury, even though your doctor tells you that your tests look fine? How does stress cause pain? This book will give you a fundamental understanding of movement as a mind-body process. You can use this understanding to get the maximum benefit from any form of exercise you choose, while minimizing the risk of injuring yourself.

This knowledge can also be of tremendous value in the arts. When you think of movement arts, you likely think of dancing. But most arts are movement arts, because you create the art by moving your body in some fashion. Playing the violin, painting, and ceramics, for example, all depend on movement. If an artist improves the economy of body movement, his or her technique will improve. By the same token, an artist putting unnecessary strain on various body parts risks eventual injury. I have worked with a number of young musicians who have sustained serious physical injuries early in their careers as a result of poor movement techniques. By integrating neuromuscular retraining into artistic training, many unnecessary injuries can be prevented and the development of technical expertise can be accelerated.

Muscular Retraining for Pain-Free Living is divided into two sections. Part 1 of this book provides a conceptual understanding. Once you have read this part, you will have an understanding of the importance of body awareness in musculoskeletal functioning, the role of movement patterns, how your body compensates for pain and injury by altering your muscle tone and skeletal alignment, and the effects of your emotional well-being on your musculoskeletal system. All of these things are related to being present, and they are all supported by your awareness of yourself in the here and now.

Part 2 of the book provides the exercises you will need and the experiential and practical application of the concepts explained in part 1. Please resist the temptation to start on the exercises until you have finished reading part 1. After reading part 1 you will better understand the essential components of each exercise so that you can approach it properly, with your full awareness.

You don't need to believe in any specific philosophy to benefit from the information and exercises presented in this book. The more you are able to observe and feel how you move and use your body, the more sensible the concepts in this book will become. It makes no difference whether you are young or old; the starting point is the same. You use movement and your kinesthetic sense in the present to unravel the pains, injuries, and musculoskeletal compensations rooted in your past.

It generally takes adults longer to make neuromuscular changes than it does children, because an adult's muscle habits are much more ingrained. However, I have worked with adults over seventy who learn just as fast as teenagers, showing that age is not the determining factor here; rather, it's how in tune you are with your own movements. Much of the interference with easy and pain-free movement comes from muscle habits that you have accumulated over your lifetime. Many people mistake the accumulation of habits and poor kinesthesia for the aging process itself, but these are two separate issues. The less stuck you are in your muscle habits, the easier change will be for you. To begin to get unstuck requires an awareness of what your body is doing and how it feels.

Underlying all the therapeutic exercises I teach is awareness. I have found a way to base an effective musculoskeletal therapy on kinesthetic awareness. The exercises and techniques I have developed and use are helpful for correcting body use, alignment, and muscle tension. The principles presented in this book can be used in any sport or physical exercise and in any endeavor involving human movement. The sky is the limit.

PART ONE

The Basics of Body Pain

I

Presence of Mind, Presence of Body

> Each moment is a place you've never been.
> —*Mark Strand*

PRESENCE OF MIND means to be aware of what is happening in the present moment; presence of body means to be aware of your body in the moment. When you are really living in the moment, your experience of yourself includes actual feelings from your body, not just a bunch of ideas and memories from your mind. In other words, your awareness of your body in that moment influences your sense of what you are in that moment. A more specific term to describe body awareness is *kinesthetic awareness* (or kinesthetic sense), which literally means your sense of movement. Kinesthetic awareness is the key to solving many pain problems and is the subject of chapter 2.

Your kinesthetic sense gives you the feeling of being "embodied," of being three-dimensional and part of what is around you. Take a look around at our sedentary, mechanized, fast-paced culture, and you will see that many of us are living lives that are far from embodied. We take our corporeal selves for granted. Many people spend most of their time sitting down. Their minds are working, thinking, or seeing, while their bodies are sitting (or slouching) in a foam-padded seat. How many people do you know who really work with their hands and/or bodies? We now have machines that do much of the physical work that people used to do themselves. We also have cars to transport us, so most people have to make a special effort to go walking during the day. Our muscles have tightened up from the stress of living this way and don't move normally even when we exercise. The fact is that the more we live in a man-made environment, primarily urban or suburban, the more potential we have for becoming "disembodied." Our muscle and joint sensors are not stimulated enough, so we gradually stop feeling them. This lack of kinesthetic awareness and our disembodied lifestyle can result in muscular pain.

Awareness facilitates healing. Awareness can *be* healing. The relationship between them has generally been overlooked in conventional approaches to health and medicine. Awareness is a function of the body and the mind together—that is, the whole person. A change in awareness is a change in your nervous system, which in turn is a physiological change.

You can use your capacity for awareness to make positive changes in your musculoskeletal system (your muscles, tendons, and joints) to reduce pain. Your body awareness, specifically your kinesthetic awareness, can improve how your muscles function. Muscles function because they are connected to nerves. The nerves tell the muscles what to do and how to do it. *Muscular retraining* involves using awareness to change the way muscles behave.

Let's take a quick look at a few concepts that relate to using awareness for muscle retraining.

Process and Goal

When you apply yourself to any activity, whether it is an exercise or anything else, you can approach it with either a goal orientation or a process orientation. To be goal-oriented is to remain focused on a definite outcome or destination that you choose at the beginning of the endeavor. Climbing Mount Everest so that you can plant your country's flag at the summit is a good example of a goal-oriented endeavor. To be process-oriented is to focus on *how* events unfold along the journey. Hiking up a mountain so that you can enjoy the physical exertion and the sights, sounds, and smells of nature along the way is an example of process-oriented behavior. If the climber in the first example does not reach the mountain's summit, the endeavor has failed. The hiker in the second example, on the other hand, benefits regardless of whether he reaches the top or not. *Process,* then, refers to your actual moment-to-moment experience in the present. *Goal* refers to the outcome you hope to achieve. If you are pursuing an activity with a goal, such as running around the block, your process —how you accomplish it—might change every second, even though your goal remains fixed throughout.

We all have the capacity for awareness, and our awareness affects our physiology. When awareness is part of a therapy, that therapy becomes somewhat process oriented. This is because our awareness, like any process, is always changing.

In my practice, I incorporate movement exercises and techniques with a process-oriented approach to achieve the goals of pain relief and flexibility. This process is kinesthetic. Increasing your kinesthetic awareness will help your neuromuscular system begin to function more efficiently, which causes pain to decrease and flexibility to increase. In this case, the goal (pain relief) is achieved by focusing on the process.

Employing a process-oriented approach to accomplish a goal is something of an art or a balancing act. Underlying the success of this approach is the understanding that you cannot force a process to happen how and when you want. By forcing your way toward a goal, you interfere with the process itself. For example, you cannot force yourself to relax because once you do, you are, by definition, tense. Think of the art of navigating a sailboat. You have a destination—a goal—that you want to reach, but to reach that destination you have to go with the flow of the wind and the current. The wind and current are not within your control, but if you work with them, you can use their power to go where you wish.

The Goal of Learning

Goals are essential in life because they give direction. Of course, regardless of how determined you are to reach your goal, you have no way of knowing what will happen along the way. If you rigidly adhere to a goal, you may miss something new and valuable that is opening up right in front of you.

While you are in the process of learning something new, you don't really know what you will learn ahead of time. Genuine learning always involves dealing with the unknown. If you are open to the process, you can learn from anything and everything, whether you are traveling to a new place, making a new friend, moving your body in a new way, or simply staying home to watch television. Every breath you take is new, as is every cloud that traverses the sky and every bird that hops on your lawn. *Learning is a state of mind.*

When you make learning your goal, you solve the problem of being too goal oriented, because you can never learn all there is to know. Learning is the perfect goal because it can never be fully achieved.

Restraining Versus Guiding

If we were watching a surfer ride a wave, we might marvel at the way he maintains balance. He could be balancing by *restraining* his body, by forcing muscles to hold on tightly. This restraining might give him a feeling of control because his goal-oriented mind is attempting to dominate his body. Or he could be balancing by *guiding* himself to move with the wave. The guidance comes as a result of relaxing and being aware of the here and now, the actual process of balancing. As you might suspect, restraining your muscles ultimately makes them inflexible, whereas guiding your muscles keeps them flexible. The following example illustrates the two types of control and the differences between them.

I have worked with many young musicians who play with unnecessary tension in their arms and hands. This tension eventually causes them severe pain. In the course of correcting their problems, they invariably realize that they have been trying too hard to control their hands, a habit that often begins early in their musical training. Their playing technique, which allowed them to play increasingly more difficult pieces as time went on, also increased the tension and force in their upper bodies. In other words, they controlled their movement by restraining their muscles. To solve their pain problems, these musicians had to learn how to release unnecessary tension and use their kinesthetic awareness to guide their movement without restraint. They learned that it is far more practical to use awareness and relaxation than restraint, because it minimizes the pain.

The moral of this story is that, when pursuing a goal, you can fixate on the end point, tighten up your muscles, and force your way through, or you can become aware of the moment-to-moment process and patiently guide your body along the path of least resistance.

Awareness and Concentration

A distinction can be made between *awareness* and *concentration*. These words generally refer to paying attention, but they actually have very different meanings. In simple terms, awareness involves widening your scope of consciousness, while concentration involves narrowing your scope of consciousness.

When you concentrate on something, you are using effort to prevent yourself from being distracted by extraneous input. This creates a narrow focus. In contrast, awareness allows you to focus without any mental effort.

The value of awareness is exemplified in many Eastern philosophies. The ancient Chinese sage Lao Tzu said, "By doing nothing, everything is done," advising people to allow life's events to occur without forcing particular outcomes. When you use awareness, your mind allows a flow of events to occur; when you concentrate, your mind tries to force the direction of events in a certain way. Most of us are trained to use concentration by narrowing our focus of attention. This is contrary to what Lao Tzu proposed.

For example, many things happen in your mind and body when you play the piano, and all of them affect how you play. If you concentrate on your fingers to the exclusion of everything else, you will not notice the strain that you place on your arms, shoulders, and possibly your entire body. It may seem like a simple matter to broaden your awareness to include your whole body, not to mention

your heart and mind, but to do so you have to let go of your familiar way of controlling yourself. For many, this is the most difficult
part of retraining.

Becoming Aware of What Is Actually Happening

Once when I was showing a friend one of my exercises, he told me
that I was using the same approach that his painting teacher used in
his class. His teacher asked the students to experiment with the way
they used their vision, to only see the colors and shapes of what was
in front of them, without thinking in terms of familiar objects with
particular names. When something is named, it is defined, and that
definition can limit a person's ability to see it fully and without pre-
conceptions. The painting teacher was helping his students see the
colors and shapes that were really in front of them.

Our senses tell us what is really happening. You must use your
senses to listen to music, to taste food, to feel your emotions, to communicate with others, and to feel your body. Experiencing life as it
actually is, in the now, is fundamentally different from experiencing
life through a veil of ideas about how it once was or how you think
it should be.

This subject applies directly to muscular retraining. Most of my
clients do not sense their movement and posture accurately. This is
typical of most adults. They usually think they sense their movement
clearly, but when they start to use my exercises and techniques, they
realize they were wrong. Over time, they have become increasingly
out of touch with their kinesthetic awareness. When I ask them to
describe specifically what they sense when they move, they will tell
me what they *think* is happening, not what they *feel* is happening.
This is because they are not actually feeling their body, they are thinking about it. They will describe a vague sense of their own movement, which is mostly based on their memory of how movement
feels, not the actual feeling in the present moment.

For the benefit of your entire musculoskeletal system, you need to
have accurate kinesthetic awareness. Ideas about how you think you
are using your body or how you think you *should* be using your

body are of little value if you cannot sense what is actually happening as you use your muscles. You cannot force your kinesthetic awareness to return quickly or simply take a pill to have it return to normal. Regaining your awareness is a learning process.

EXPLORATION 1

Lie flat on your back. Notice that there is a space between your lower back and the floor. This is the natural curve, or arch, of your lumbar spine (see illustration 5.2 on page 85). Slowly bend your knees so that your feet are flat on the floor. As you are doing this, feel how your pelvis changes position and your lower back becomes flatter. Repeat this a few times, until you can clearly feel the difference in the position of your pelvis and lower back when your legs are straight and when they are bent.

Now, lie with your knees bent and your feet flat. Intentionally increase the curve in your lower back, making sure that your tailbone stays on the floor. Can you feel your lower back muscles working to increase the lumbar curve? Notice the direction in which your whole pelvis moves when the lumbar curve increases.

Next, move in the opposite direction by pressing your lumbar spine down into the floor and raising your tailbone. To do this, the back muscles you were using previously need to relax, and your abdominal muscles need to engage. Specifically, your rectus abdominal muscle presses your lower back into the floor (see illustration 5.4 on page 88). Place your hands on your abdomen; you will be able to feel this muscle push outward as it tightens. When the rectus abdominal is tight, it flattens out the arch in your lower back.

Alternate a few more times between increasing the arch in your back to feel your back muscles work and pressing your lower back down to feel your abdominal muscles work. When the lower back muscles work, the abdominals relax and vice versa.

2

Kinesthesia: The Sixth Sense

> The foot feels the foot when it feels the ground.
> —*Buddha*

THE FIVE SENSES of sight, sound, touch, smell, and taste give you information about your body and the world around you. Dark or light, hot or cold, loud or quiet, sweet or salty, hard or soft—all of these stimuli are discerned through your senses. The kinesthetic sense, or *kinesthesia,* is the sensory information that comes from muscles, joints, and movement. Kinesthesia is typically considered a part of the sense of touch, but because it is so vast in and of itself, I like to think of it as our sixth sense.

Kinesthesia is from the Greek words *kines* ("movement") and *aisthesia* ("feeling"), literally "movement feeling." It is your internal sense of your body and enables you to sense what your body is doing at any given time. Your sense of muscular effort, tension, relaxation, balance, spatial orientation, distance, and proportion are all qualities of your kinesthetic awareness. These different facets of kinesthesia are so ordinary, yet so essential to your bodily sense, that you may well take them for granted. Just like your other senses, your kinesthetic sense developed in the early stages of life and simply became part of who you are. It is essential to your musculoskeletal system. It is also invisible. Perhaps that is why it is often overlooked as an important health factor. But its effects can be seen in your posture and your level of muscular tension. Musculoskeletal pain, even severe pain, can result from habitual muscle tension, from poor posture that causes tissue compression, from muscular reactions to physical impact (such as a car accident), or from unresolved emotional stress. Increasing your kinesthetic awareness can help unravel and resolve all of these problems because you need to be able to sense your body accurately in order to move it comfortably. Again, you need to be able to sense, or feel, your body accurately in order to move it comfortably. Kinesthetic awareness is the basis of my work with people.

Your nervous system senses environment: your body, your emotions, your thoughts, and the entire world around you. Your nervous system takes it all in through your senses. The more you can sense, the more open you are to information.

The Kinesthetic Sense

Your kinesthetic sense informs your brain of the whereabouts of your body. Kinesthetic receptors are nerve receptors found in your muscles, tendons, and joints. Your brain takes information from these receptors, processes it, and forms perceptions about position, shape, effort, tension, relaxation, and direction of movement. Your brain does this continuously, creating what amounts to an ever-changing kinesthetic awareness, much like a sensory picture. This picture gives you the awareness of how a part or the whole of your body feels at any given movement—the position of your limbs, the tension in your shoulders, the distance between your feet and your waist, whether you are standing up or lying down, and so on. For example, if you close your eyes and raise your arm, the kinesthetic receptors in your body will tell your brain what is happening. Your brain forms an impression that your arm is up. Without the kinesthetic sense, you wouldn't know where your arm is, because your eyes are closed.

If you would like an example of what is meant by kinesthesia, try this. Sit with your arms at your side and your hands resting in your lap. Slowly raise your right shoulder toward your right ear. Can you feel the muscles in your neck and the top of your right shoulder as they engage to raise your shoulder? Keep your shoulder up for about 10 seconds. Slowly lower it, and notice how the feeling of muscle effort changes in the right side of your neck and shoulder as your shoulder goes down. When your shoulder is nearly back to its usual position, stop and keep it still for another 10 seconds. You are still using your neck and shoulder muscles, but with less effort than before. Now raise your right shoulder toward your ear again, lifting it as high as you can. Notice whether your left shoulder has risen also. Relax your left shoulder muscles completely while your right shoulder is raised. Feel the difference of effort between your right and left shoulder muscles. Now relax your right shoulder. Check again to find whether there is a difference in the way your right and left shoulders feel. Even though both sides are relaxed now, the right side might feel a little looser than the left because you just increased your kinesthetic sense by paying attention to the feelings of effort and relaxation in your muscles.

Whether we know it or not, we depend on our kinesthetic sense to provide reliable information so that we can use our bodies properly. Consider what happens when your feet "fall asleep" after your legs have been in the same cramped position for too long. Have you ever tried to walk when your feet were asleep? It's not easy. Your feet feel stiff when you walk on them, but if you sit down and move your feet with your hands, you discover that your feet are not actually stiff. Walking is difficult because your brain cannot adequately sense your feet and therefore cannot properly tell your muscles what to do. Even though you have been walking for most of your life, the memory of walking alone does not provide your brain with enough information to make the process smooth and easy. Your brain also needs continuous, new kinesthetic information to enable you to execute your movements smoothly. Your brain guides your muscle movement, while the kinesthetic information continuously supplied by the kinesthetic receptors guides your brain.

Take another example. Imagine that you're bending to pick up a box from the floor. When you begin to pick it up, you get a feel for the box's size, shape, and weight (resistance to movement). You use this kinesthetic information, probably without even realizing it, to determine how best to lift the box. You sense the weight of the box, and you apply physical effort in proportion to the expected weight. Now imagine what would happen if you thought the box weighed fifty pounds, when in reality it weighed only five. Your brain would prepare your muscles for the effort of lifting fifty pounds. When you lifted the box, you would apply too much effort and might lose your balance as a result.

Many people think that muscle control comes from strength, but strength is actually secondary to kinesthesia. Muscle control requires coordination and guidance, which come from the kinesthetic sense. If you're skiing, for instance, you must remain balanced while twisting and turning at high speeds. Your brain relies on kinesthetic and visual input to tell your muscles how much to shorten or lengthen at any given moment, thereby keeping you balanced. If you have good muscle strength but poor kinesthesia, your coordination and ability to guide your body within space will be poor despite your strength.

Kinesthetic Awareness

Your kinesthetic receptors are working all the time. Even though you are aware of only a fraction of the information they constantly communicate, your brain takes it all in and processes it, almost entirely below the level of awareness. When you walk, your brain uses all of the available kinesthetic information to guide your movement, but there is such an enormous volume of information being communicated at such a high speed at every moment that you could not possibly be aware of it all. What you notice is the information that is strongest or most relevant at any given moment.

For the most part, then, your kinesthetic sense functions automatically. This is natural and normal. Have you ever been driving a car, with your mind on something other than how you are driving, and suddenly found yourself at your destination with little recollection of how you got there? You might not remember stopping at traffic lights, passing other cars, or making the necessary turns from one street to another. How did you manage this without having an accident? The visual and kinesthetic input continues to enter your brain even when you are unaware of it. The movement patterns of driving to a familiar location are so deeply ingrained in your neuromuscular system that you can automatically process and use the sensory input to control the body movements necessary for driving, as if you were a sophisticated robot.

Although your kinesthetic sense is able to function without any intentional help from you, you can intentionally use kinesthetic input to improve the skill of your movement. This is otherwise known as "paying attention." Imagine that you are walking on a trail that goes along the side of a hill, where the ground beneath your feet is slanted to the right. Your kinesthetic sense continuously picks up the information that your left leg does not straighten as much as the right, that you are leaning a bit to the left, that your feet are not level, and so forth. If this kinesthetic input is strong enough, you will feel that the ground is slanted beneath your feet. Since you can feel the slanted ground, you can intentionally alter the way you use your legs and feet to adjust to the slope and guide your movement. Although it may be possible to walk for hours and be unaware of what your body is doing, as in the earlier driving example, if you pay attention to what you are feeling, you are less likely to stumble because your brain is better informed about what is happening. This means that the better your kinesthetic awareness, the more stable and safe and relaxed you will be when you move.

Under normal circumstances, attention is free-floating and tends to pick up an arbitrary and changing array of kinesthetic input. Even though you cannot possibly notice all of your body's kinesthetic sensations in a single instant, it is natural and healthy to be able to notice specific areas of your body if your attention is focused there. For instance, I may not notice the toes of my right foot curling as I write this sentence, even if they have been doing so for a long time. But if someone points out to me that I am curling my toes, I ought to be able to focus my attention on my right foot and feel that I am tensing my foot muscles. This may seem simple and obvious, yet many people are not able to sense their kinesthesia clearly.

Kinesthetic Dysfunction

The kinesthetic sense can become so distorted that an individual cannot accurately sense where his or her body is in space or whether muscles are engaged or relaxed, even when attention is focused directly on them. This condition is not the result of neurological damage, but rather of learned insensitivity to kinesthetic input. F. M. Alexander calls this phenomenon "debauched kinesthesia," while Thomas Hanna refers to it as "sensory-motor amnesia." I refer to it as *kinesthetic dysfunction,* because it is literally a dysfunctional kinesthetic awareness. Kinesthetic dysfunction is the inability to sense your kinesthesia accurately, even when you intentionally attempt to pay attention to it. In my professional experience, I have found that problems with kinesthesia are an extremely common cause of muscular pain, yet most people are unfamiliar with this connection.

If you have kinesthetic dysfunction, you cannot accurately sense whether certain muscles are relaxed or engaged. As a result, tensed muscles remain tense, and sooner or later the tension becomes painful. As long as your kinesthetic awareness is dysfunctional, you cannot correct the way you carry and use your body.

If you find that your body is becoming more and more stiff and inflexible as you get older, you may be mistaking a steady increase in habitual muscle tension caused by a decrease in kinesthetic awareness for the inevitable aging process. If your kinesthesia is dysfunctional, you may also mistakenly conclude that pain is the result of a mechanical problem in your body, such as a torn muscle or arthritis, when there is no actual mechanical problem at all. If your kinesthesia is dysfunctional and you are injured, you will have more than the expected number of muscular reactions to the injury, and you may end up confusing the painful effects of these reactions with the pain of the injury itself.

Kinesthetic dysfunction is not caused by nerve damage, nor is it an injury. Rather, it is a problem with how you *perceive* the messages coming from your kinesthetic receptors. You need two things to correct kinesthetic dysfunction: new sensory input and a willingness to pay attention to it.

How the Kinesthetic Sense Becomes Dim

Whenever you experience continuous, constant, and unvarying sensory input for a prolonged period of time, your perception of that input will be altered. You can find many examples in daily life of how your nervous system adapts to repetitious and continuous sensory input. You may not notice the sound of your own refrigerator, even if it's a noisy one. Your nervous system adapted to the constant sound long ago. In other words, you got used to it, and when that happened, you stopped noticing the noise. If the refrigerator noise suddenly stopped, you would probably notice the quiet immediately because of the sudden change in sensory input.

During a family vacation in my childhood, we passed through a small factory town en route to our destination. I remember this town because it was permeated with an overwhelming odor of sulfur, the smell of rotten eggs. When the odor first hit me, I was nearly gasping for air in the backseat of the car. I can remember looking at all the people in town and wondering how they could possibly tolerate the terrible smell. They were all walking around without disgusted expressions on their faces, as if nothing unusual was happening. We stopped for lunch in that town and stayed for a couple of hours. In this brief amount of time, without realizing it, I became accustomed to one of the worst odors I had ever encountered to the point where I no longer noticed it. As we drove out of the town, there was a point at which I suddenly noticed that the smell of the air had changed back to normal. We had driven out of the invisible sulfur cloud.

Becoming accustomed to a strong odor or getting used to the noise of a refrigerator are examples of how the nervous system tends to stop noticing repetitive and monotonous input. Another example of this is when you put your shirt on in the morning. At first you are clearly aware of the shirt against your back. After a short time, however, you probably don't notice the feeling of the shirt any longer because the input from the skin sensors in your back has become constant, with little variation.

Getting used to the feeling of the shirt on your back is innocuous, but getting used to unvarying kinesthetic input can be harmful to your health and well-being. Constant and unvarying kinesthetic input often comes from muscles that are constantly tensed and joints that are constantly compressed. After some period of time, you get used to this input, become insensitive to it, and lose awareness of what is happening in your body.

From Dim to Dysfunctional

I said earlier that your brain handles your kinesthetic sense automatically. If it is automatic, why does it matter if your kinesthetic awareness is diminished in some areas? Because when you cannot *intentionally* sense kinesthesia, your neuromuscular system does not *automatically* sense it properly either. If this is the case, your brain will be unable to guide your muscles to relax correctly. For example, if you cannot accurately sense your abdominal muscles, then these muscles will not be activated properly during exercise or when you stand and walk. And because these muscles are not being activated fully, you could easily mistake your condition for muscle weakness.

I have treated hundreds of people whose neuromuscular systems were incapable of fully accessing and using the muscles they could not sense clearly. Through the repetition of kinesthetic input due to constant muscle tension and a lack of variety in movement, the neuromuscular system can lose its ability to activate and use the muscles efficiently. Your neuromuscular system requires accurate kinesthetic perception to use your muscles properly. It is not known exactly how kinesthetic dysfunction occurs, but it certainly does occur. When kinesthetic perception is dysfunctional, the neuromuscular system cannot properly execute muscle control or create balanced muscle tone.

Dysfunction of this sort commonly occurs in people with chronic muscle tension from pain reactions, injuries, inefficient body alignment, or prolonged psychological stress. This condition is completely invisible. It cannot be detected with x-rays, magnetic resonance imaging (MRI), blood tests, nerve conduction tests, or strength tests. Kinesthetic dysfunction can only be discovered by asking a person if he or she can perceive the effort and relaxation of muscles and then testing whether this perception is true to what the muscles are actually doing.

Since kinesthetic dysfunction is, by definition, a lack of awareness, you don't know it is happening because you can't feel it. How can you notice something that you cannot feel? This is the fundamental predicament of kinesthetic dysfunction: you don't know why you have muscle pain because you cannot sense the degree of effort that your muscles are constantly making.

The Role of Kinesthetic Dysfunction in Muscular Pain: Hal

I can recall when I first began to suspect the pervasive role of kinesthetic dysfunction in muscular pain. I was working with a client named Hal, an active thirty-year-old with pain throughout his upper back along both sides of the spine. His physician told him that he probably had ankylosing spondylitis, a degenerative spinal condition in which vertebrae gradually fuse together. A blood test revealed that Hal had a certain factor in his blood that is typically present in people with this condition. Although not everyone with this blood factor has ankylosing spondylitis, his physician told him that his symptoms and test results made it a likely diagnosis. Hal simply refused to believe that he had a degenerating spine. A different physician told him that the problem might be in his muscles and that therapy might be able to help him, so he made an appointment with me.

Hal had the personality of a real go-getter. His mind was quick, and his movements were fast and efficient. During his first session, I began teaching Hal corrective movements. He performed the movements exactly as I instructed him, all very rapidly. I asked him if he could feel his back muscles working, and he said that he did. He also said he thought it was obvious that he could feel his muscles working. He told me that he had been an athlete his whole life and that he had been a runner before his back pain became too severe. I dropped the subject and taught him a few basic floor exercises involving the use of his back and abdominal muscles.

At his next appointment a week later, Hal told me that he felt no better. In fact, he thought the exercises might have caused his back to hurt more. He said that this did not bother him; exercise always hurt his back, and he did not mind a little pain. I told him the corrective exercises were intended to be painless. I explained that exercises are painful when muscles tighten instead of release at the proper time. His pain increase made me think that he might have been pushing too much through the exercises. I asked him to go through all of the exercises while I watched him closely.

Hal performed the exercises with precision, exactly as I had showed him. I asked him again if he could sense effort in his back muscles when he used them and relaxation when he stopped using them. He replied with some exasperation, "Of course I can." I found it puzzling that he didn't get at least temporary pain relief from the exercises.

I asked him to repeat one of the exercises one more time. It struck me that he was moving rather quickly, so I asked him to repeat it as slowly as possible. When he slowed down, I could see that his back muscles were not completely relaxing between each movement, a necessary aspect of that particular exercise. I then asked Hal to intentionally relax his muscles for a few seconds after each movement. After trying the exercise again slowly, he said that his back would not relax right away and that it took a number of seconds before he could sense his back muscles letting go. I asked him to wait patiently until his back muscles completely relaxed before proceeding with the next movement. This slowed him down considerably.

At this point, something changed in Hal's awareness. He said that he could now feel his movements much more clearly. In fact, he said that even though he thought he had been feeling his movements before, he could now tell that he had barely felt them at all. Hal had *assumed* that he was relaxing his back muscles and thus could not understand why I was emphasizing feeling the relaxation so much. Within a few minutes, Hal's range of motion doubled on the back extension exercise he had been doing. He said that his movements felt less jerky and more controlled than before. He stood up at the end of our session and declared that his back was no longer hurting.

I saw Hal a few more times to teach him more corrective movements and alignment techniques. He said he was able to start aerobic exercises again and his pain was no longer a problem. By chance, I saw Hal running along the beach about six months later. He ran up to me with a big smile on his face. The first thing he told me was that he still did the exercises I taught him every day. He also said that he could run again, just like before, and that he had no more back pain.

I like to understand why things happen, and I could not simply attribute Hal's improvement to good luck. Something remarkable had happened, and he and I both knew it. But what exactly had occurred? Hal's range of movement improved suddenly, but we cannot say that he became stronger because his back muscles could not have doubled in strength in a matter of minutes. Hal's relief from chronic back pain could not have been the result of stretching because the relief came while he was engaging and releasing his back muscles, not while he was stretching. Besides, Hal had done back stretching exercises for months before he met me, and they had not improved his condition in the least.

What was different about the exercises he did with me? The main difference was in *how* he did the exercises. The way Hal performed the exercises actually affected his kinesthetic awareness for the better. By moving slowly, he was compelled to pay attention to what he was doing and to move with more intention than usual. Since moving this way was very different for him, new information was sent from his kinesthetic receptors to his brain. This new and different kinesthetic information allowed his neuromuscular system to access his back muscles more effectively, which accounted for the sudden increase in his range of motion. The change in his kinesthetic awareness had changed his back.

My experience with Hal and countless other clients transformed my way of looking at recurring muscular pain. I suspected that good kinesthesia might be the result of moving well, the way a well-trained dancer or athlete does. From Hal and others like him, I learned that good kinesthesia is also the cause of moving well. In other words, good kinesthesia is both the cause and the result of proficient movement. Because good kinesthesia causes muscles to perform with skill and efficiency, improving kinesthetic awareness is an effective method for alleviating the muscular tension and pain caused by unskillful and inefficient muscle use. Many of my clients have rid themselves of recurring musculoskeletal pain by increasing their kinesthetic awareness in the specific area of pain.

Experiencing the Sense of Effort

You do not need to resort to black magic to find out if you have kinesthetic dysfunction in a particular muscle group. A knowledgeable practitioner can determine the accuracy of your kinesthesia by having you deliberately make a movement that activates a certain muscle group and then asking you what you feel. The practitioner evaluates your awareness of the effort your muscles make when they engage and the noneffort they make when they disengage.

Here is an example. I once worked with a woman named Helen who had recurring lower back pain. To assess her kinesthetic awareness of her lower back muscles, I had her lie face down on an exercise mat and lift her right leg, which required the use of her lower back muscles. I could see that Helen was both lifting her leg and engaging her lower back muscles. I asked her if she could sense which muscles she was using to perform this movement. She could not sense any effort in her lower back muscles. I touched her back with my hand and asked if she felt any effort there. She said she did not. To make sure she knew what I meant by *effort,* I asked her where she felt a sense of effort. She replied that she could sense effort in the back of her hip area and the backs of her thighs, where muscles were also being used. Clearly, Helen knew what I meant by *effort,* but she simply could not feel it in her lower back muscles.

Helen became upset when she realized that she was incapable of doing something that seemed so incredibly simple. She told me that she would not have given much thought to it if I hadn't made such a "big deal" of it, but now she was starting to worry. I told her that her inability to sense her back muscles was a very big deal if she ever wanted to stop having back pain, but there was nothing to worry about because it could easily be corrected. Helen quickly regained her normal kinesthetic awareness by using the floor exercises and alignment techniques I taught her. After eight appointments with me, her back pain was gone and she had gained the awareness to prevent its return.

I have observed countless cases of kinesthetic dysfunction. Sometimes it has been causing problems for years and can be corrected in a matter of minutes via a movement awareness exercise or a hands-on technique; sometimes the correction can take many weeks or months. But I have never worked with anyone who wanted to regain normal kinesthetic awareness and didn't.

Kinesthetic Dysfunction: Case Studies

Some people think that kinesthetic awareness is so simple and basic that it can't possibly be the answer to a complicated pain problem.

Sometimes it is the entire answer, sometimes it is part of the answer, and sometimes it is not the answer at all. Because kinesthetic awareness is simple and basic, it is fundamental to any musculoskeletal issue. It makes sense to regain healthy kinesthetic awareness first, before going through complicated treatment procedures that overlook its importance.

The following examples show three typical clients with kinesthetic dysfunction. Kinesthetic dysfunction is not a rare condition related to unusual problems. On the contrary, it is frequently involved in common muscular pain, as in the lower back, neck, and hips.

The Pain Cycle: Steve

Kinesthetic dysfunction is part of a typical cycle of recurring pain: high muscle tension leads to pain; pain leads to restricted movement; restricted movement leads to kinesthetic dysfunction; kinesthetic dysfunction leads to poor muscle use; poor muscle use leads to higher muscle tension, which causes more pain; and so on. Any of these can be the starting point for the pain cycle, which perpetuates itself indefinitely unless interrupted. Increasing kinesthetic awareness is the key to interrupting the pain cycle.

Steve's case shows the whole pain cycle in action. Steve was thirty-four years old when he came to see me. He had constant high muscle tension and pain in his lower back. Since he had hurt his back years before while playing high school football, Steve assumed he had a bad back and would simply have to live with it. He didn't exercise like he used to, because exercise caused his back to hurt more. He didn't realize that he held his entire waist in a rigid position no matter what movement his body made. Steve's muscular rigidity had developed gradually, so he could no longer remember how his hips and waist used to move. Because he moved his waist so little, he no longer experienced the sharp, jabbing pain he once had. Instead, he felt a constant tightness and ache.

Because his back muscles were always engaged and his waist movement was so limited, Steve's brain was not getting the necessary variation of kinesthetic input. The input from his back muscles varied little because they were constantly tight, whether he was raking leaves, climbing stairs, or sitting at a desk. His nervous system had adapted to this constant, monotonous kinesthetic input by diminishing his sense of muscle effort; Steve had kinesthetic dysfunction. He couldn't accurately sense what was occurring in his lower back muscles. All he could sense in his lower back was pain and stiffness. Since his brain needed accurate and varied kinesthetic stimuli to know what to do with his muscles, he was not able to use his muscles correctly. His back muscles were not engaging and releasing normally when he moved. They were tense and remained so throughout the day.

Steve's kinesthetic dysfunction had impaired his ability to access and use his back muscles. Without realizing it, he had recruited other muscles to help him compensate for his stunned back muscles. These other muscles were not meant to move his hips and waist efficiently, so they soon tired, which caused further pain. Eventually, Steve felt the pain spreading beyond his lower back to these other muscles. The increase in pain caused his back muscles to contract even more, making his back even more rigid and increasing the kinesthetic dysfunction.

Steve was going around in a cycle of tension, pain, and kinesthetic dysfunction. How could he break out of this vicious cycle? When I watched Steve closely, I could see that he moved his hips and waist as if they were all one inflexible piece and that he never twisted from the waist. He habitually and constantly contracted all of the muscles that would otherwise move his hips and waist. I recommended that he begin by dealing with the kinesthetic dysfunction. I systematically taught him exercises and alignment techniques, which he practiced every day on his own. Steve soon began to realize that the very areas where he felt pain were areas with constant muscle tension and fatigue. That tension and fatigue cause pain may seem obvious, but there is a big difference between knowing something intellectually and being kinesthetically aware of it. Steve knew that he had tension, but because it was only an idea in his mind, it did not help him. He could not feel his continuous muscle effort, and therefore his muscle pain and tension did not change. Periodic massage and chiropractic treatments decreased the pain and made his life much more bearable, but they did not address the underlying kinesthetic dysfunction, which Steve did not even know existed until he came to see me.

After twelve sessions with me and conscientiously doing exercises on his own, Steve told me that pain was no longer running his life. He broke the cycle by retraining his muscles to relax. He said that he had not been to the chiropractor for more than a month and did not expect to ever need him again. He was happy to take care of his back himself.

Fear of Pain: Edith

Sometimes a painful accident or injury can make you so afraid of having more pain that you try to ignore your body as a way to escape. This is what happened to Edith, whose car was rear-ended while she was waiting to make a left turn. She had severe neck and right arm pain for months after the accident. X-rays and an MRI showed no structural damage to her skeletal system. When one of her physicians told her that she might have arthritis, she went to a specialist who told her that there was no arthritis in her shoulder or neck. He correctly diagnosed the pain as muscular and sent her to see me.

During her first appointment, I had Edith lie on her back and asked her to let me gently move her head without any muscular effort on her part. No matter which way I moved her head, she would unintentionally push it against my hands. When I asked if she could sense that she was pushing against my hands, she said she couldn't.

I sat at Edith's right side and began slowly moving her right arm. I asked her to relax her arm and allow me to move it for her. Again, she unconsciously resisted any movements I attempted. I asked Edith if she felt relaxed, and she said, "I think so." This was a clue that her kinesthetic sense was dim, since I had asked her what she *felt,* and she replied with what she *thought.* I then asked her to close her eyes, and with my hands under her arm, I raised it to about a forty-five-degree angle, so that her hand and elbow were well off the treatment table. I could feel that she was doing all the work of lifting her arm, so I slowly removed my hands. Like magic, her arm remained suspended in midair. I asked Edith if her arm still seemed relaxed, and she said it did. I then asked her to open her eyes and look at her arm. To her surprise, her arm was off the table. She had no clue that her arm muscles were tensed. Her kinesthetic awareness was so dysfunc-

tional that she needed her eyes to confirm that her arm was not resting on the table. Because her kinesthetic awareness was so unreli-
able, she could not use her neck and arm muscles properly or relax
them. If Edith's kinesthesia had been functional, she would have
been able to relax these muscles voluntarily.

Prior to seeing me for treatment, Edith had no understanding of
kinesthetic awareness and kinesthetic dysfunction. She had no idea
of her own potential to solve her problem by regaining her natural
awareness and control of her muscles. She assumed that someone
else was going to step in and solve her problem. But because of her
kinesthetic dysfunction, her condition remained unchanged and the
treatments she received had no effect.

Edith had two interrelated problems: kinesthetic dysfunction and
a lack of understanding. Kinesthetic dysfunction can be changed
with corrective exercises and learning to become aware of the body's
movements. She placed the responsibility for restoring her well-
being on the doctors and therapists she was seeing. Because she was
not kinesthetically aware, she could not take responsibility for her
own healing. She told me that her problem was a burden and she just
wanted to get on with her life. I told her that her awareness *was* her
life and she could only get on with it by being where she was. Of
course, she didn't like where she was—in pain—and wanted to be
somewhere else. I did not expect her to enjoy being in pain, but she
needed to get back inside her body and regain her kinesthetic awareness if any treatment was going to be helpful.

Edith soon realized that she had been afraid to let herself sense
her upper body movement since the accident because she thought it
might make the pain worse. This fear prevented her from doing the
one simple thing that would help her get better—regain her kinesthetic awareness. She made the important discovery that feeling pain
and feeling tension are two different things. Without realizing it, she
had been avoiding pain by ignoring her bodily sensations altogether,
which cut her off from her kinesthetic awareness. When she felt her
movements, she found that she was able to control the muscles that
had been involuntarily contracted ever since the accident. At this turning point, her pain began to decrease. Eventually, Edith enjoyed a full
recovery.

Kinesthetic Awareness and Age: Bob

Kinesthetic awareness is something that we tend to take for granted. As children, we explore our environment and develop our kinesthetic sense by moving our bodies. Movement is important for children because it creates a wide range of kinesthetic input, such as balance, muscle effort, spatial orientation, and coordination. This input becomes the foundation for movement awareness that persists throughout our lives.

I have observed that younger people generally have better kinesthetic awareness than older people. However, I have also seen exceptional cases of children with astonishing kinesthetic dysfunction and octogenarians with excellent kinesthetic awareness. Whether kinesthetic dysfunction is the result of injury, poor posture, emotional stress, or something else, it becomes familiar and habitual if unchecked. The longer you live with these habits, the longer it will take you to break them. People often mistake the inflexibility that comes from the accumulation of habits for the natural decline of old age. Obviously, our bodies do age. But aging is not a purely physical event; the role of awareness should not be ignored in the aging process. Since your potential for kinesthetic awareness does not age, you are never too old to improve this awareness to increase flexibility and decrease pain.

I met Bob when he was eighty-five. He had experienced constant lower back pain for many years. His stride had gradually been reduced to a hobble. When he stood up, he was bent over at the waist, and he told me that he was unable to stand up straight.

Even though he had been an athlete in his younger days, Bob was completely unable to feel either his abdominal or lower back muscles. In the front, back, and sides, his waist was locked up tight. Years of recurrent back pain had caused him to limit his movement more and more and to tighten more and more muscles. Moving his pelvis became impossible because he lacked kinesthetic awareness there. He could no longer feel that his pelvis was a movable part of his body. Were it not for the pain in his back and hips, he would probably have forgotten they existed.

At Bob's first therapy session, I had to help him down to the exercise mat on the floor. With considerable repetition and guidance from my hands, he began to perform a basic waist exercise. After forty-five minutes of repeating the same simple movement, Bob was still struggling and seemed to be getting nowhere. He could not feel what his muscles were doing. Since he could not sense his waist movement, he had to take my word for it that I was not asking him to do the impossible.

Suddenly, as if out of the blue, Bob could feel the effort in his lower back muscles. The difficult movement immediately became easier. Bob was absolutely thrilled when he felt his pelvis begin to move without pain. He told me that he could not remember the last time he'd felt his body move this way. I suggested that he practice the corrective exercise at home three times a day.

Two weeks later, Bob came back. He was standing visibly taller and walking with much longer strides. He told me that his back hurt less than it had in years and he could now get up from a chair without a shooting pain in his back. His wife, who had come with him, said Bob was so excited about the changes in his body that he was doing the corrective exercise more than three times a day. He had even figured out a modified version of the movement that he could do while sitting in a chair, which he did intermittently throughout the day.

Bob got down to the floor mat at his second appointment without any help. He was able to sense the muscular effort, relaxation, and motion in his abdominal and back muscles clearly. He moved his hips and waist with confidence that pain would not result. We went over some new, more challenging corrective movement exercises. When Bob got up unassisted from the floor mat, he looked me in the eye and said that for years he had gone to all kinds of people for his back pain, and I was the first person who ever helped him.

Bob's rapid progress after only one visit was due to the fact that his efforts in that session began to reawaken his kinesthesia. His enthusiastic practice at home speeded up the process. This was the first therapy that had made him feel better, because this was the first therapy that made him *feel*. Prior to his first session with me, he was incapable of properly using any of the back exercises that he had learned from various physical therapists and doctors because he literally had no sense of what he was doing. Nonetheless, he was able to regain his kinesthetic awareness after all those years of pain and rigidity.

A Physical-Mental-Emotional Interface

Kinesthesia is an interface between the body, the mind, and the emotions. Not only is it of tremendous practical value for correcting the movement patterns that control muscle tension, it also provides the link that explains how emotional stress leads to musculoskeletal pain.

Suppose you are sensing tension in a hip muscle. Your mind perceives the kinesthetic sensations that originate in your body. If you sit quietly and focus attention on that muscle, you should be able to observe both the physical sensation of muscle tension and the mental perception or awareness of the hip tension. Yet there is only one experience happening—the experience of you sensing your hip. So is sensing physical awareness or mental awareness? It is both. The body and mind are not separate.

Imagine that you are feeling nervous about a job interview, and you notice a sensation of tightness in your abdomen. That tightness is the kinesthetic sensation of your muscular reaction. If you focus attention on the sensation in your abdomen, you can become more aware of both the muscle tension there and your emotional feeling of nervousness. This is because your body and mind are not separate.

Kinesthetic awareness allows you to know, accept, and experience your emotions. To experience an emotion, you must be able to feel your body; therefore, the most direct way to get in touch with your emotions is to be kinesthetically aware of your body. Tension between the eyes, pain and stiffness in the neck and shoulders, a feeling of expansion in the chest or a sinking feeling in the stomach, jittery legs, or pain just about anywhere are physical sensations that can occur as part of your emotional experience at any given time. We will see in chapter 6 how some muscle tension and postural habits result from continuously triggered emotional reflexes. Kinesthetic awareness can help to relax these muscles. It can also help you become aware of the emotional reactions that led to your muscular and postural habits.

A kinesthetic experience is also an emotional experience, so forgetting kinesthetic awareness is an effective way to suppress or deny uncomfortable emotions. Suppressing kinesthesia happens when you intentionally try to hold back an emotion. For example, if your feelings are hurt but you don't want to cry, you can suppress your kinesthesia by thinking of something other than your actual feelings, while at the same time tightening the muscles of your face, neck, shoulders, abdomen, and other areas. Thinking about something other than what you are actually feeling takes your attention away from the bodily sensations that are part and parcel of feeling hurt. Tensing the muscles interrupts the kinesthetic experience of sadness and makes it easier for you to think about something else. I am not recommending this because habitual suppression of kinesthetic and emotional experience is not only emotionally unhealthy, but it can also cause bodily pain (more about this also in chapter 6).

Kinesthetic awareness affects your physical and emotional flexibility. These two types of flexibility are not separate; they support one another. When your kinesthetic awareness is clear, you can experience your feelings as they occur. Essentially, this means you know yourself. As a result, you are more flexible in dealing with stress and better able to make choices about your life circumstances.

Kinesthetic awareness should be incorporated naturally into exercise programs and athletics, beginning with physical education in schools. For this to occur there needs to be a fundamental shift in how we perceive ourselves. We would need to understand the importance of kinesthetic awareness, to stop being disembodied people and become embodied people. To an embodied person, kinesthetic awareness is an ordinary part of life. The most extraordinary thing about it is that so many people don't have it. The problems that result from this lack can also be extraordinary.

Kinesthetic awareness affects your level of muscular relaxation, movement coordination, and emotional well-being. The greater your kinesthetic awareness, the more enjoyable any kind of movement will be for you.

EXPLORATION 2

This exploration is to improve your kinesthetic awareness of the transverse abdominal muscle, which wraps horizontally around the back, sides, and front of your entire abdomen (see illustration 5.4 on page 88).

Lie on your back with your knees bent and your feet flat. Place your hands on your abdomen. Pull your belly in toward your spine, and notice how your abdomen feels under your hand. When you engage the transverse abdominal, you will clearly feel your abdomen pulling in, *away* from your hand. To be sure that you are using the right muscle, do not allow the length between the front of your pelvis and your chest to become shorter as you pull in your belly. If it does, you are using the rectus abdominal muscle (also shown in illustration 5.4). The transverse will pull in when it is isolated, whereas the rectus will press out.

If that part of the exploration seemed easy, you can try something a bit more challenging. Think of your transverse abdominal muscle as having an upper and a lower section, each with a different function. Stand up and lean your back and pelvis against a wall, with both knees bent slightly and your feet about ten inches from the wall. First, pull in the lower half of the muscle, just above your pubic bone. You will feel your lower abdomen pull in and press the back of your pelvis into the wall. Next, pull the upper half of the muscle (around and above your navel) in and up. You will feel your chest lift a little and your lumbar spine push into the wall. Your back muscles remain completely relaxed as you do this so that your back stays flat against the wall. Repeat this slowly until you can distinguish the difference between the lower and upper parts of this muscle.

3

Movement Patterns

Great things are not done by impulse, but by a
series of small things brought together.

—*Vincent van Gogh*

LEARNING A NEW MOVEMENT SKILL can take a tremendous
amount of attention at first, but after the learning takes place, you can
do it without thinking. Remember what it was like when you first
learned how to swim, use a sewing machine, drive a golf ball, type,
or drive a car. Driving a car with a standard transmission requires a
certain timing of the arm and leg movements. Initially, this timing
can be very challenging. But eventually, with practice, you can perform these movements while listening to the radio, talking to your
passengers, or thinking about something else—your feet and arms
shift the gears and steer without you thinking about it.

Even the simplest movement, such as raising your arm, is the
result of innumerable processes within your nervous system that
organize and coordinate your movements. The muscles, bones, and
other tissues provide the structural support for movement, while the
nervous system orchestrates the use of this support. The nervous system feels what is happening in your body as it directs the muscles in
their actions.

Memory, a process of the nervous system, is essential to learn a new
movement activity. When you learn to ride a bicycle, for example, you

acquire memories of how it feels, such as the sensations of using your arms, pedaling, and losing and regaining balance. In the process of learning to ride, your nervous system uses the information from your errors to develop ways of executing the activity successfully.

When you have learned a new activity, you can easily and automatically perform an action that you could not perform previously. For example, you are suddenly able to balance on a bicycle. At this point, the neurological and muscular processes related to cycling are consolidated into a memory of the action as a whole. This consolidated memory is known as a *movement pattern*.

Once you learn how to walk, you can do it automatically. When you get up in the morning, you can jump out of bed and begin walking right away without any practice, because your movement pattern for walking has already been established. If you did not develop movement patterns, you would have to relearn all of your movement activities every day.

Because you learn movement patterns through experience and trial and error, there is no guarantee that the movement patterns you learn will be effective. Injuries, emotional stress, congenital defects, and nutrition can all affect both the way you move and the way your movement patterns develop. If you learn to play the violin in a relaxed and supportive environment, you will likely develop movement patterns different from those you would have if you learned to play in an environment full of pressure and dread. You may end up learning to play the violin in either case, but the movement patterns you develop will reflect the tension that you experienced in your mind and your muscles while you were learning to play.

If your movement patterns are effective, you will enjoy an economy of motion, with a minimal amount of strain and tension. Movement is possible because of the coordination of your nervous and musculoskeletal systems. The musculoskeletal system receives messages from the nervous system and performs the movement. However, if these two systems are not well coordinated—because of a painful injury, emotional stress, or repeated use of the body with improper skeletal alignment—movement patterns become dysfunctional (more about this later in this chapter).

How Movement Patterns Develop

Let's take a look at a simplified example of how movement patterns develop. Imagine that a six-year-old girl is riding a bicycle for the first time. Since she has never been on a bike before, she has no memory of how it feels to ride one. When she first gets on the bicycle, she is unfamiliar with the feeling of keeping her balance. Her brain records and organizes the details of the kinesthesia related to maintaining and losing her balance every time she tries to ride.

The next day she tries again. Her brain automatically retrieves the memories of how she felt while maintaining and losing her balance the day before. The kinesthetic information now in her memory combines with her current kinesthesia. Her brain uses all this information to help guide her in her current attempts to balance on the bike. The clearer her kinesthetic impressions are now, the clearer her kinesthetic memory will be on subsequent attempts.

On the third day, she gets on her bicycle again. After a few more attempts, she can ride without falling. Gradually, the kinesthetic information has become sufficiently organized in her memory to allow her to successfully balance on the bike. On the first two days she persevered, yet she still could not balance. Today, she can get on and ride easily. She now possesses a reliable kinesthetic memory of the muscle activity and coordination required for a sense of balance. This kinesthetic memory is a movement pattern that automatically guides her each time she gets on her bicycle.

In some ways, a movement pattern is like a sewing pattern. If you want to sew five shirts, you can design one pattern for a shirt and simply follow the same pattern for all five. Since you have a reliable pattern, you do not need to think through the design of each shirt you sew; you can simply follow the original pattern. Movement patterns are similar: once you establish a pattern of muscle activity and body movements, your body can use the pattern over and over.

All of the failures you encounter when you are first learning a new activity gradually guide your brain toward a more efficient way of organizing and coordinating the movement. By experiencing what does *not* succeed, your brain eventually determines what *does* succeed. Some failure is necessary to successfully accomplish anything. A movement pattern is the result of successful actions that get the job done.

Since movement patterns work automatically, you don't need to think about the activity for which you have established a movement pattern in order to perform that activity successfully. The movement pattern for cycling automatically takes care of the complex neuromuscular coordination required for balancing. You can put your attention elsewhere. You can look at the scenery without being concerned about falling over.

Generally speaking, when you reach the point at which you automatically use a movement pattern for an activity, we say that you have "learned" that activity. In actuality, however, learning is not an end point at which you eventually arrive, but rather a series of stages that are part of an ongoing process of acquiring information and using that information to refine your skills and improve your performance.

If you are a beginner at the piano, you cannot play a Mozart sonata because your movement patterns are not developed enough to play anything that complicated. If you attempt to play the sonata, your attention will be occupied by trying to play all of the notes. However, a concert pianist, who has practiced so much that the movement patterns of his hands are finely honed, can play the notes effortlessly and focus on other aspects of the sonata, such as emotional interpretation of the music.

The Organization and Disorganization of Movement

Your musculoskeletal system is made up of many different parts that need to work together in order for you to move. The extraordinary levels of organization and economy of movement that your system achieves are possible because of movement patterns.

For movement to be organized, movement patterns must function in a way that makes sense. Imagine that you hear a bird chirping and you want to see that bird. Your eyes will immediately move to find it. If the bird is behind you, your head and spine need to turn to allow your eyes to see the bird. This happens automatically, so you may take it for granted. Your body is programmed to organize your movement so that your head and spine move in a way that lets you see what you want to see. The organization of your movement allows you to carry out your intentions.

The fact that movement patterns work automatically is an advantage. You use movement patterns every day. Indeed, you could not even begin to function without movement patterns. When you stand up, you don't need to remind your leg muscles to engage. Thanks to your movement patterns, your leg muscles engage when you stand, even if your attention is on the yellow finches at the bird feeder. Otherwise, you would fall over.

When a movement pattern causes muscles to work too hard or to remain lax when they need to engage, movement becomes more strenuous and less efficient and produces more tension. This is what I call a *dysfunctional movement pattern (DMP)*. A simple way to think of this is as a bad habit of muscle use.

An example of a DMP is when a person habitually tenses her neck muscles every time she inhales. You don't need to tighten your neck muscles to breathe. Nonetheless, many people do this as a matter of habit. This habit is a DMP. The result can be a stiff neck.

A DMP can be difficult to change because it feels so familiar. For instance, if you habitually stand with your upper body far behind your central balance point and I use my hands to guide you to a more balanced alignment, you might feel like you are leaning forward. This is a commonplace initial experience for many of my clients, so I ask them to look in the mirror to verify that they are really standing vertically rather than leaning forward. Many people tell me that balanced alignment feels strange to them at first. The familiarity of DMPs can make them resistant to change, despite the fact that they may be causing pain.

A DMP may or may not be troublesome to you. If your habit of how you hold a spoon does not follow proper etiquette, you may not be bothered. On the other hand, if your DMP results in the overuse of your spinal muscles every time you stand up, you could be bothered quite a bit. DMPs cause you to use your body in a tense and damaging way, which can lead to hardened muscles, tendon strain, and cartilage degeneration.

Influences on Movement Patterns: Sarah

The major factors that influence the development of your movement patterns are the basic movement patterns you learn in childhood, the influences of specific movement training, injury, muscular reactions to pain, repeated postures (occupational and otherwise), and emotional stress.

In childhood, you form patterns for all of your movements. You learn to sit, walk, run, use your hands, and so forth. Genetics control the development of many of these patterns. Environmental influences—your observation of other people's movements, your physical activities, and the emotional support you receive—also play a major role in determining your movement patterns.

A friend left her toddler-age granddaughter at my house one afternoon so that my wife and I could look after her. When I was walking down the stairs with this little girl, I noticed that she had a very unusual way of swaggering from side to side as she walked. I held her hand tightly because I was concerned that she would lose her balance, but she never fell. *They don't call them toddlers for nothing,* I said to myself. Almost a year later, I met the mother of this little girl. I was walking behind her, when something made me think, *Have I seen that gait before?* Then I remembered walking down the stairs with her daughter. The mother had the same way of swaying from side to side. This idiosyncratic walking style was a custom-made movement pattern. By the age of one, the child had already developed the same pattern as her mother.

Some people are quick to assume that their DMP—as well as the resulting poor posture and pain—are genetic. Many people believe that they inherited back problems from a parent who also had back problems. It is usually impossible to know for certain if a DMP is genetic or learned in childhood. Although genetics are obviously a big factor, this explanation can be an easy excuse to dodge personal responsibility for changing habitual behavior. It is generally most effective to assume that your DMP has been learned. The good news is that because many DMPs are learned, they can be unlearned.

A clear example of this was a twelve-year-old girl named Sarah. When I first began working with Sarah, she had constant left hip pain. Her hip pain was occasionally so sharp that she could barely stand up. Sarah was very athletic. She played one team sport after another, all year round. Since chronic muscular pain is unusual in someone Sarah's age, she went to a sports medicine physician who diagnosed her condition as left hip epiphysitis (abnormal development at the end of the bone). Sarah's family physician suggested that she see me for muscular retraining.

Sarah was fairly limber and had no restriction in her range of motion. I was unable to recognize anything unusual about her movement patterns until I studied her posture while she was standing still. Sarah would only stand with all of her weight on one leg or the other. Her feet were both turned out (duck-footed, or laterally rotated). She looked relaxed and comfortable in this position.

I asked Sarah to stand with her feet parallel to each other and put equal weight on both legs. She was able to do so, but every five seconds or so she would lose her balance and begin to fall backward. Her arms would shoot up reflexively to help her catch her balance. Sarah did her best to hide the fact that she was losing her balance, but the more I watched her, the more obvious it became.

I asked her to try to keep her balance in the new position, but she was unable to do so. Then I asked her to return to her typical way of standing. When she did, her weight shifted to one side or the other, and she could stand indefinitely without losing her balance. Only when she stood in an anatomically neutral and balanced position did she lose her equilibrium. I asked Sarah to walk and noted that she took very short strides. Although she was not aware of it, taking short strides was her body's way of compensating for the overall instability of her alignment.

I asked Sarah's mother if she had ever noticed her daughter's difficulty with balance, and she said that neither she nor anyone else had ever noticed or mentioned it before. I asked Sarah if she knew that she had trouble balancing. She replied that since she never stood with her hips and feet in a parallel position, she had no idea. Given that she excelled athletically, no one would have suspected her of having a problem with balance.

Sarah's balance problem was due to DMPs in the muscles near her waist, the body's center of gravity. Despite her athletic ability, flexibility, and strength, Sarah was unable to perform a number of simple exercises with ease. These included muscular retraining exercises that used her abdominal, back, and hip muscles in a way that was totally unfamiliar to her. She had no kinesthetic awareness of what I was asking her to do, and as a result, she could not access those muscles properly.

I taught Sarah a number of muscular retraining exercises, which she practiced every day. By the third appointment, the constant hip pain was gone, but her ankle had begun hurting a little. By the fifth appointment, Sarah had no pain at all in either her hip or her ankle. At her sixth and final appointment, Sarah was able to maintain her balance easily for five minutes with her feet in parallel (neutral) position. Sarah's father then told me he noticed that she was running differently and looked more relaxed. I asked if she was taking longer strides, and he said that she was. I had never suggested to Sarah that she take longer strides; it happened automatically when her balance improved.

Prior to her sessions with me, Sarah was not aware of her DMP. Standing with distorted hip and leg alignment felt normal to her. Taking short strides, despite her long legs, was also normal. As so often happens, Sarah had become accustomed to her own DMPs.

Using muscular retraining exercises that increased her kinesthetic awareness and her ability to access all of her muscles, Sarah was able to establish new movement patterns that gradually corrected her balance. She had previously attempted to stretch and strengthen her legs and hips, but that did not address her kinesthetic dysfunction or her DMP.

Sarah's hip pain was due to chronically contracted hip muscles compensating for her lack of balance control at her body center. The brain does whatever it can to maintain the body's balance, even if it means locking up the hip and lower back muscles, as in Sarah's case.

Sarah's ankle and knee pain resulted from the constant strain of using her legs with such a tight, restricted hip.

As I worked with Sarah, I often wondered how she had developed such a distinct way of avoiding the use of the muscles around her body center, especially as she had done so much running and playing in her life. One day, when Sarah's mother came to my office, I watched her walking with her two canes. I could see that she also lacked the support of the muscles in the waist area for keeping herself balanced and upright.

Sarah's mother had multiple sclerosis, a gradually developed neurological condition in which nerve impulses cannot be conducted properly through the nerves. One of the symptoms of this disease is some loss of voluntary control of many skeletal muscles. She was only partially able to use the muscles of her body center to support her alignment and movement.

Out of curiosity, I asked Sarah's mother if I could watch her do a few basic movements involving her waist muscles. She had the same unusual movement patterns as Sarah. In the mother's case, these patterns were the result of the degenerative process of multiple sclerosis. Sarah did not have multiple sclerosis, yet she had developed muscle use patterns similar to those of her mother. Sarah's ability to initiate a change in her body use after only two months demonstrated that her muscle problems were learned and habitual.

Because Sarah was twelve years old, she was easily able to improve her kinesthesia and her muscle use. If she had come to see me at age forty-eight, her DMPs would have been much more ingrained and would therefore have taken longer for her to change. She would have had another thirty-six years of compensating for hip, ankle, and knee pain by shifting her alignment farther off center.

When an adult begins to deal with pain caused by DMPs from earlier in life, he or she often discovers a cascade of different muscular habits, each one compensating for previous habits. The good news is that by increasing your kinesthetic awareness and reinforcing functional movement patterns, you can gradually undo the effect of years of compensation. After all, a DMP is really just memories. With new kinesthetic awareness, habits can be changed at any age. The process you go through is no different at forty-eight than it is at twelve. But you need to be realistic; changing your DMPs is going to take some time. Basically, the better your kinesthetic awareness, the faster you can change DMPs.

Dysfunctional Movement Patterns Resulting from Pain and Injury: Judy

Physical injury can also lead to a DMP by activating protective muscular reflexes. A reflex is an automatic muscular response, as with a protective reflex in response to pain or a balancing reflex in response to the change in position of muscles, tendons, or bones (see chapter 4 for more about reflexes). If a reflex remains activated long after an injury happens, the affected muscles eventually develop a DMP. Here is an example of this common circumstance.

A forty-year-old woman named Judy came to see me because of back pain that started a few months after she had broken her left ankle in a hiking accident. The x-rays showed that her bones had healed normally, yet she was still walking with a limp months after the cast had been removed. Immediately after the cast was removed, her ankle felt stiff, but Judy said that the pain was minimal after a few weeks. Still, she continued to walk with a limp. She also noticed a new development: lower back pain on the right side. The back pain persisted for several months before I first saw her. Judy's friends told her she was still limping, but she was not always aware of it. She wondered if the limp and the back pain had anything to do with each other.

Without knowing it, when Judy began to walk with a cast on her left leg, her gait became uneven—she limped—because she could not bend her left ankle. To compensate for the lack of left ankle motion, she shifted some of her weight to her right leg and tightened the muscles in her left hip every time she took a step. Her pelvis was tilted, so that it was higher on the left side than on the right. During the six weeks that she walked around with a cast on her left leg, Judy developed a DMP in her hip and lower back muscles. When the cast was removed, she continued to limp because this DMP remained in operation.

By using the simple muscular retraining exercises I taught her, Judy quickly regained a clear kinesthetic sense of her hips and lower back, improved her walking pattern, and eliminated her back pain.

A limping gait is a visible sign of a DMP. However, many DMPs that result from injury or pain may not be obvious initially. I have seen hundreds of cases where a person had unknowingly altered his or her muscle use after an injury or mishap, but no significant pain symptoms appeared for years after the accident. The way one's body compensates for an injury may not be dramatic enough to cause strain and pain immediately. Yet years of living with a DMP can eventually put undue strain on the muscles, ligaments, cartilage, and connective tissue.

Dysfunctional Movement Patterns Resulting from Repeated Motions and Postures: Amy

Postures and movements that are repeated constantly or frequently over a long period of time can also lead to DMPs. A good example of this phenomenon can be seen in the Charlie Chaplin movie *Modern Times*. Chaplin is working in a factory where he has to repeat the same arm movements to turn a wrench all day long. One day, his arm movements become unstoppable, and he walks out of the factory like a robot, attempting to use his wrench to tighten anything that looks like a nut.

If you hold a position for a long time, you can develop a DMP in much the same way that repetitive muscle use can. This is because both stationary postures and repetitive motions involve continuous muscle use. An example of this is arm pain among people who spend long hours at a computer keyboard. Even though typing at a keyboard may not seem physically strenuous, the constant muscle use can create a DMP. If you stretch and change positions frequently, you can ward off this muscle dysfunction, because any movement variation changes the kinesthetic input, which in turn relaxes the habitual muscle tension.

Amy provides a striking example of how a fixed posture and repetitive muscle use can cause DMPs. Amy was sixteen years old when she came to see me and had played the violin since early childhood. For a number of weeks before coming to me, she had been experiencing severe left arm and hand pain whenever she played her instrument. She had reached the point where she was unable to play for more than a few minutes before the pain forced her to stop. She also had lower back pain on the left side.

I asked Amy to stand and face me. Her face and torso were facing toward me, but her hips, legs, and feet were turned to the right. In other words, her waist was twisted to the left. The more I looked at her, the more clearly I could see the twist in her waist, as if she were standing to play the violin. Her posture had conformed to the asymmetric position she assumed when playing her violin. As a result, she had DMPs in her entire upper body. Amy had no idea that her waist twisted when she stood up. When I asked her to intentionally stand in a symmetrical position while looking in a mirror, she said she felt twisted to the right. Even when she looked in the mirror and could see that she was not twisting at the waist, she still felt as though she was. This bizarre experience of the eyes saying one thing and the body saying another is a common one in my office. Amy's kinesthetic awareness was incorrect because it had conformed to the effects of years of DMPs in her waist, back, and shoulders.

Amy had not learned to play the violin with relaxed arms and shoulders. The left arm and hand pain she felt while playing occurred because her left shoulder was nearly immobilized with tension. The left shoulder was pulled down and held still by many of the same muscles that were twisting her waist. These muscles were also causing the pain in her lower left back. It was as if there was a taut, invisible cable running from her left lower back up the left side of her torso and down the back of her left arm, all the way to her left little finger. All of the muscles all along this invisible cable were tense. When she played the violin, the taut cable pulled on her left arm and hand, which was why they hurt.

After six sessions of hands-on therapy and retraining exercises, Amy returned to playing the violin without pain in her shoulder and arm. Her lower back pain was also gone. Because her movement patterns were so ingrained, she needed to continue doing the exercises daily so the old DMPs did not come back.

I have seen many adult musicians who felt pain like Amy's. Some of them played with pain for many months before it became too much to bear. Because they waited so long to attend to the problem, not only did they have to deal with their original DMPs, but they had also developed muscular tension from compensating for pain and inflexibility for so long. Ingrained DMPs such as these can take months or years of dedicated practice for a person to change. Fortunately for Amy, her doctor suggested treatment only several weeks after the pain began interfering with her ability to play the violin, so the problem was solved quickly.

Dysfunctional Movement Patterns Resulting from Emotional Stress: Phil

Emotional stress can trigger muscle contractions, which can eventually become a DMP. In Phil's case, his emotional state was affecting his back muscles.

Phil was forty when he came to see me with severe pain in his middle and lower back. He had had the pain for a number of years and had reached the point where sitting was so painful that he could barely drive his car. In the past few years, different doctors and therapists had told him that his pain was the result of misaligned vertebrae in his spine, weak back muscles, and gallbladder malfunction. Phil had tried chiropractic treatment, physical therapy, and gallbladder surgery, but the pain continued.

When I first saw Phil, his poor posture was the first clue that his back muscles were working overtime. The natural curve in his lower back was greatly exaggerated, which put unnecessary strain on his lower back muscles and joints. I had Phil do a variety of movements involving his lower back muscles. Phil had kinesthetic dysfunction in his lumbar muscles, so he could not feel the effort in his lower back when he used those muscles. But he had no problem feeling the pain in his lower back. I worked with him until he became kinesthetically aware of his back muscles, so that they functioned evenly on the right and left sides. I taught him corrective exercises to do daily, with specific instructions about where to focus his attention during each exercise.

When I saw Phil a week later, he told me that the pain was half what it had been the week before. He had finally been able to finish a remodeling project in his home, something he thought his back would never allow him to do. Now that he could feel the tension in his back muscles, he was able to begin to relax them. The constant muscle tension in his back was now obvious to him, whereas before, all he could feel was pain. He now understood the important difference between feeling pain and feeling muscle tension.

In another week, Phil said that he could clearly feel how certain stressful situations throughout the day were causing his back muscles to contract; he noticed his back tightening up and returning to its habitual exaggerated posture. If the tension were severe enough, he would feel the familiar stabbing pain in the right side of his back. He noticed this response specifically when he was feeling frustrated and angry.

Phil's pattern of reacting to stress and personal problems with anger went hand in hand with his DMP, which involved so much muscle tension that muscles would spasm and cause back pain. A muscle spasm is a strong, painful, involuntary muscle contraction (more about this in chapter 4). In Phil's case, the spasms were an automatic muscular response to the habitual emotional upset he had experienced for many years.

Phil and I discussed the differences between suppressing anger, feeling anger, and expressing anger. He later discovered through experience that when he gave himself the space to simply feel angry without suppressing it or venting it on someone or something, his back pain would subside. The kinesthetic awareness he regained in his back muscles gave him immediate biofeedback about the state of these muscles and his emotional well-being. Not only did Phil learn how to change his movement patterns, he began to change his emotional patterns as well.

Movement Patterns and Skilled Movement

Increasing your skill at a movement activity, whether it's shooting hoops, performing surgery, or driving a car, involves using your kinesthetic awareness to develop increasingly efficient movement patterns. As a general rule, the more efficient your movement patterns, the less energy you expend and the easier an activity is to do. Using more than the minimum muscular energy necessary to perform an activity is therefore essentially a waste of energy. For example, have you ever noticed how professional hockey players make skating look so easy? They skate with an economy of motion, which makes their movements clean and graceful.

You can learn some movement skills by practicing on your own, but other skills require or benefit from a movement teacher. A movement instructor—anyone involved in athletic or artistic instruction—needs to have good movement patterns, because that teacher is a role model for his or her students. It is the teacher's job to help students develop efficient movement patterns to increase their skills.

If you are fortunate enough to have a skilled movement teacher, you can bypass many potential problems. A good teacher will make sure that you learn to use your body correctly. As a result, you will avoid developing DMPs that interfere with your progress and, worse, lead to injury or pain. Ideally, anyone who teaches movement skills to athletes and performers should emphasize the importance of kinesthetic awareness and relaxation.

I once taught myself how to play the flute. After five years of playing for my own enjoyment, I had my first flute lesson. My instructor taught me techniques in the first lesson that I would have taken years to discover on my own, if I ever did. After a few weeks, I realized how much easier playing would have been if I had started lessons five years earlier. I would have benefited from the teacher's twenty years of experience in playing and learning.

In addition to limiting your skill at an activity, a DMP puts you at greater risk of injuring yourself by causing strain in the muscles and other soft tissues of the body. As in Amy's case, musicians frequently injure themselves this way. Playing an instrument requires you to repeat the same actions frequently. The repetition of movement is not necessarily a problem, but it becomes a problem when a DMP is involved.

Musicians, athletes, and other performers run into two general sets of movement pattern problems. The first results from the specific techniques they have learned for using their body, such as holding a guitar or using their wrists and hands at the piano. If these techniques inherently produce strain, then the musician constantly reinforces techniques that can cause injury. The second set of problems results from habitual tension, both physical and emotional. If a musician experiences mental duress while learning to play an instrument, all of his muscles will be tense when he uses them to play. The pressure could be the result of simply trying too hard, of a parent or teacher being overly demanding, or of feeling pressure to succeed and compete with others. Pervasive tension can cause problems of tendonitis, nerve entrapment, and joint damage, all of which can end a performer's career.

Athletes, like musicians, are susceptible to these problems as well. If a runner has an asymmetrical gait pattern, the strain of maintaining that gait may cause injury. If you have an asymmetrical gait but are not a runner, you may never develop a problem. But if you are an athlete who is repeating the same motions over and over, any imbalances are amplified.

I once saw a nationally ranked track star who had difficulty running because of constant pain in her shinbone. Her doctors were debating whether she had a stress fracture in her leg. By asking her to perform certain movements, I was able to demonstrate to her that, stress fracture or not, her leg strain and pain were the results of a DMP in her hip muscles. She needed to change the way she used those muscles to be able to run without pain.

Repatterning Your Dysfunctional Movement Patterns

You can repattern a DMP through muscular retraining, a process that involves moving in a new way. The trick is to combine kinesthetic awareness with comfortable, nonforceful movements. Many people have been trained to think of exercise as something that is naturally painful, forceful, and arduous. This attitude does not work for muscular retraining exercises. In fact, muscular retraining involves moving as easily as possible by avoiding the use of any unnecessary muscles.

Effort and Ease

The word *effort* comes from the French word *esforcier,* meaning "to force oneself." Forcing suggests using more effort than is absolutely necessary. The more skilled you are in movement, the less force you need and the more relaxed you can be. Even though classical ballet is one of the most demanding physical disciplines, a great ballerina can make her movements look easy, almost effortless. Graceful movement involves using physical effort so economically that it neither appears nor feels forced.

It is a commonly accepted sign of mastery when a performer makes a difficult art appear easy; this occurs when the performer is relaxed with what he or she is doing. I once saw a performer in the circus who was able to ride a unicycle on a rope while tossing seven teacups and saucers one at a time onto his head, stacking them on top of each other. He even tossed the final teacup up with his foot! This magnificent performer made a seemingly impossible act look easy, without the least bit of strain or anxiety showing in his face. What he did, of course, required years of practice, but because he was relaxed, his body was working at its best.

I once discussed effort and mastery with Seung Choi, a tenth-degree black belt who founded the martial art of *choi shin do.* Seung mastered martial arts at a young age, and over a long career, he had trained a number of world champions in kickboxing. He said that relaxation is the key to becoming skilled at kickboxing and grappling (similar to wrestling). These sports require a tremendous amount of energy, and on the surface, they may not appear to have much to do with relaxation. In fact, the opposite is true. Seung's point was that when a person is relaxed, his mind does not interfere with what his body needs to do, so the reflexes are sharp and the body moves efficiently. He emphasized that relaxation is not a state of sleep, but rather a state of heightened self-awareness. He considered relaxation to be fundamental not only to the martial arts, but to life in general.

The ideal way to move is to "go with the flow" of the movement, rather than forcing yourself. Although it sounds simple in theory, it's not necessarily easy in practice. Why should it be? The mastery of a physical skill would not be noteworthy if it were easy. The challenge of mastering a physical skill is not in conquering your own body, a piece of equipment, or a technique. Instead, it is in developing the ability to use the least amount of effort necessary to accomplish your goal. You must learn how not to interfere with your own movement. For this, it is helpful to understand the difference between doing and nondoing.

Doing and Nondoing

You maintain your balance by using kinesthetic and visual input to guide your body. To accomplish this, your brain must process vast amounts of information, of which you are largely unaware. You may be busy talking to somebody, but your neuromuscular system is simultaneously dealing with the details so that you don't fall.

You might have the impression that *you* are doing the balancing by virtue of your attention and effort, but actually your neuromuscular system is accomplishing the task. As you know, you can ride a bicycle while paying attention to something else and your neuromuscular system still manages to keep you from falling. The interaction of your kinesthesia with your existing movement patterns organizes and maintains your balance. The "I" within you—your ego, personality, or whatever you want to call it—cannot make movement happen. Your neuromuscular system does.

Of course, you are involved in your own movement; you are not a preprogrammed robot. You are involved either by facilitating your movement or interfering with it. You can facilitate movement by *allowing* the movement to happen, rather than forcing it to happen. By being kinesthetically aware, you increase the kinesthetic input, which allows your neuromuscular system to optimize the use of your muscles. You can interfere with movement by *forcing* it to happen. The idea of making movement happen rather than allowing it to happen represents a mind-set that creates unnecessary pressure. The pressure sets you up to use too much effort and therefore makes your muscles too tense.

Here is a simple example of the difference between doing and nondoing. Have you ever found yourself doing something clumsily while other people are watching you, yet doing it easily when you are by yourself? When you are being watched, you may be trying so hard to look skillful that you get in your own way. When you are alone and not trying to impress anyone, you are likely to be more relaxed, and as a result, your body works better. I have noticed more than once while watching figure skating on television that a skater can have a terrible performance during competition, yet during the exhibition skating after the competition has ended, she skates magnificently. When the pressure is off and she is performing for the sheer enjoyment of it, without worrying about winning, she is allowing the movement to happen, not trying too hard to make it happen.

When you try too hard to make a movement, you are likely to engage a DMP. Your muscle use and overall movement will follow a preprogrammed track based on your past experience. If you want to discover a new way of using your body or performing an activity, you need to break free of your DMPs. You do this by letting go, by feeling your muscles and alignment in new ways, by coordinating your movements in new ways—and then observing what happens. You learn new movement by feeling, by being aware. You can learn to use your body with more relaxation and better alignment by feeling the differences between new and habitual ways of moving.

Just like a musician or an athlete who trains by practicing certain movement patterns over and over, you train yourself by sitting, bending, walking, and performing all of the other ordinary movements of your daily life. If you make these movements with awareness and ease, you train yourself to relax and develop functional movement patterns. If you make these movements with excessive force and tension, you train yourself to be tense and create DMPs.

Part 2 of this book presents movement exercises that you can use to change your movement patterns. These exercises work because they encourage an increase in your kinesthetic awareness while you use your muscles in a new way. All of these movement exercises are based on the way your body is naturally designed. Each suggests a potentially new way to move. With practice, these movements and techniques can teach your body how to relax, to move more smoothly, and to use less effort.

You have the capacity to pay attention to what you are doing from moment to moment. As soon as you begin to experience yourself in the present, new sensory information begins to challenge the old movement patterns in your brain. Your brain has the opportunity to alter and improve on the old patterns, which gives you the possibility of experiencing movement in a new way. You can begin to correct musculoskeletal pain problems by focusing your attention on your kinesthetic awareness. A remarkable thing happens when you become aware of the kinesthesia in a tense area of your body: you become more present, and the process of relaxation begins immediately and automatically. All you have to do is provide your brain with the kinesthesia by paying attention to what you sense, and your brain starts to work out the details. If your brain senses that certain muscles are engaged unnecessarily, it immediately begins the process of disengaging them. This is also an example of nondoing in that your attention is doing the work, and as long as you are not trying hard to make relaxation happen, it happens.

Here is a movement exploration that I often use with my clients that you can try now. If you are wearing shoes, take them off. Stand up and begin walking slowly. Notice the way your feet feel as they touch the floor. Pay attention to every point of contact between both feet and the floor. Step so that your heel touches the floor first. Does every inch of your foot touch the floor, from your heels to your toes? Does your foot feel pliable like a piece of rubber, or does it feel stiff like a piece of wood? Just before you step off each foot, do you feel the bottom of your toes pressing into the floor? Do you use your toes at all when you step off each foot? Continue walking slowly, with your attention on your feet. Now imagine that your feet are attached to your legs by tassels, so that the ankle is completely loose when you step. Allow your feet and ankles to be relaxed as you walk. Imagine that you have soft feet, like a cat, so that you can feel every contour of the ground. Do your feet resist the ground in any way when you put weight on them, or do they relax and allow the ground to support them? Keep walking slowly, feeling any or all of the things I have mentioned. Consider the idea of *allowing* yourself to walk rather than *trying* to walk. Notice how focusing kinesthetically on your feet brings you immediately into the present and how your body is a little more relaxed than when you started. If you spend a little time walking this way every day, it will begin to feel normal to have softer, more relaxed feet, and you can begin to change movement patterns in your whole body.

EXPLORATION 3

Between your lungs and your stomach is a dome-shaped muscle called the abdominal diaphragm, or simply *diaphragm*. It is like a floor just below the lungs. When the floor goes down, space in the chest cavity increases, allowing the lungs to fill with air (inhalation). When the floor goes up, space in the chest cavity decreases, pressing air out of the lungs (exhalation).

Lie on your back with your knees bent and your feet flat on the floor. As you take in a breath, relax your abdomen completely so that it fills up like a balloon. This happens because your diaphragm is pressing down into your abdomen, and your abdomen is expanding from the pressure.

Inhale once again, and hold your breath. Still holding your breath, pull in your belly by using your transverse abdominal muscles (see exploration 2 on pages 29–30). You will feel the pressure in your belly slowly move up into your chest, as if you had a ball inside of you that moved from your belly to your chest. At this point, if you relax the transverse abdominal, the ball of air pressure will move back down to your abdomen. Breathe normally a few times, and repeat this same procedure. Continue until you can clearly feel how abdominal tension and relaxation affects the expansion of your chest and abdomen when you breathe.

4

Musculoskeletal Pain: Causes and Effects

Things should be made as simple
as possible, but no simpler.
—*Albert Einstein*

MUSCLES HAVE A TENDENCY to react automatically to feelings
of strain, pressure, and/or pain. This automatic reaction is to tighten.
Ideally, muscles would react to strain and then relax when the strain
was over. Prolonged strain, pressure, or pain can cause muscle tightening that becomes habitual, creating a dysfunctional movement
pattern (see chapter 3). This is a major cause of musculoskeletal pain.
Understanding how a DMP can cause pain requires some knowledge
about how your nerves, muscles, bones, and other structural components function.

The Musculoskeletal System

Bones are the framework of the body; they ensure that when you
move, your body retains its basic shape. The boneless jellyfish radi-
cally changes shape when it moves. Your shape also changes when
you move, but the degree of change is greatly limited by your skeleton.
Bones also provide protection for the internal organs. For example,
the skull protects the brain, and the ribs protect the lungs and heart.

Bones provide a stable, relatively inflexible support for carriage and movement. Bone can be used for leverage and to minimize the effort of your movement.

Your muscles are attached to your bones and help to keep the bones connected to each other. Body movement occurs when muscles change length, thereby moving the bones to which they are attached. When you stand up, the bones of your skeleton support you. Your muscles maintain the position of your bones. Without a skeleton, standing up would be impossible. Without muscles, balance would be impossible.

Muscles are made of strong fibers gathered in lengthwise parallel bundles. Through a remarkable electrochemical process, muscle fibers have the ability to move and thereby shorten or lengthen the muscle as a whole. When the muscle is relaxed, the threadlike filaments within the muscle fibers slide freely over one another, and the muscle is at its greatest length. When the muscle is actively working, these filaments engage by hooking onto one another, which allows the muscle to temporarily lock into a variety of lengths. For example, if you raise your arm horizontally at your side and hold it still, the muscles of your arm and shoulder are each holding on to a particular length by locking their filaments together. If you relax your arm and let it drop, the filaments release from each other.

Conventional thinking tells us that muscles produce movement by shortening, or contracting. When muscle activity occurs, however, a muscle may shorten, remain the same length, or even lengthen. Therefore, when speaking of how muscles produce movement, I prefer to use the word *engage* instead of *contract*. *Engage* and *disengage* describe the essential activity of muscles, without regard to changes in muscle length. When I talk about muscle *contraction,* I am referring specifically to a muscle that is either tense due to a reflex or one that is habitually tense over a prolonged period of time. I will say more about that later in this chapter.

Your muscles are anchored to your bones by tough, fibrous connectors called *tendons*. Although made of fibers, a tendon does not have the capacity to lengthen and shorten like a muscle and therefore remains at a fixed length. In a sense, tendons are part of both the muscle and the bone to which they attach. The attachment of the tendon to the bone can be stronger than the bone itself. For example, in some severe muscle or tendon injuries, a piece of the bone itself separates, leaving the tendon intact and connected to its anchor point on the bone.

Ligaments are similar to tendons. Just as your tendons attach your muscles to your bones; your ligaments attach your bones to one another. These tough, fibrous, nonelastic connectors help to keep your bones in place. Ligaments are all over the body in the areas of the joints, where they resist the forces that tend to pull bones away from each other. A joint is simply a place where two bones meet for the purpose of movement. In the knee joint, for instance, the upper and lower leg bones meet and move with each other. Ligaments are essential for keeping the bones of the knee joint in the proper relation to each other so the joint remains stable and easy to bend.

Cartilage is a protective material between your bones and is composed of a varying mixture of fiber and firm gel. Unlike tendons and ligaments, which are designed to resist the pulling forces in muscles and bones, cartilage is designed to resist the compression of muscles and bones. If you sit on a wooden bench, you can use a cushion to resist the compression of your pelvis against the hard surface. Cartilage has a similar cushioning effect; it prevents bone surfaces from rubbing against each other and wearing down the bone. It can be found, for example, at the ends of the bones of your arms and legs, where two bones make contact. Also, each bone or vertebra of your spinal column has a disc of cartilage above and below it. The elasticity of the discs adds to the flexibility of the spine as a whole and protects each vertebra from grinding against its neighbors.

Throughout your body is a fibrous material called *connective tissue*. One type of connective tissue is known as *fascia,* which can be likened to a gigantic piece of shrink-wrap that wraps around everything, including muscles, bones, nerves, and vital organs. The fascia around muscles is called *myofascia*. When the fascia in one area is not able to move freely, the movement in another part of the body can end up being restricted also. An analogy for this would be the following: if you are wearing a tight, long-sleeved shirt that is tucked under a belt at the waist and you lift your arms over your head, you will feel the fabric of the shirt restraining your arms. Even though the shirt is caught at your waist, it will be your arms that eventually become tired. Likewise, if your fascia is restricted at your waist, it will restrain your arms.

Fascia is more flexible when it is warm than when it is cold. It has chemical properties similar to those of gelatin, which you well know turns from liquid to solid when it is refrigerated. When you "warm up" before physical exercise, the gel in your connective tissue becomes more fluid, so you generally feel looser and more flexible. Because of the increased flexibility, your body has less resistance to movement, and you are less likely to be injured.

The Nervous System

The nervous system is composed primarily of nerves. A nerve contains many individual nerve cells bundled together by connective tissue, just like a rope that is made up of many individual fibers. A *nerve cell* is a specialized body cell that can conduct an electrical current across its entire surface, carrying information from one part of the body to another. Nerve cells are the body's messengers.

The brain is made up of nerves and connective tissue and is the headquarters of the nervous system. The spinal cord, which is housed within the protective bones of the spine, is a superhighway of nerves that shuttle information back and forth between the brain and the outside world. The brain and spinal cord together are called the *central nervous system* because they are along the central axis of the body.

The remainder of the nervous system is made up of *peripheral nerves,* which connect the central nervous system to everything else. For instance, the sciatic nerve is a peripheral nerve that connects your spine to your foot, while the ulnar nerve connects your spine to your hand. *Sensory nerves* are peripheral nerves that send information toward the central nervous system, like a highway going into a city. At the ends of sensory nerves are little receptors that pick up specific information from your body and the environment. For example, some sensory receptors in your hands detect tension in the muscles, others detect temperature, and others detect pressure on the skin. *Motor nerves* are peripheral nerves that send information away from the central nervous system, like a highway going out of a city. They are called motor nerves because they *motivate* action, meaning they carry instructions to muscles that cause the muscles to move.

Muscle Function

If you follow any motor nerve from the spinal cord out to its end point, you arrive at a muscle. The electrical message that travels through the nerve is capable of triggering a series of chemical changes in the muscle. These changes in turn produce mechanical changes in the muscle, which cause the muscle to work. As I mentioned in chapter 1, the combination of the nervous system and the muscles is known as the *neuromuscular system,* the intelligence that guides and controls movement.

Muscles follow the instructions of the nervous system. If an electrical impulse from a motor nerve is strong enough, the muscle will engage. If the nerve message stops, the muscle disengages and relaxes. A muscle cannot engage without a directive originating somewhere in the nervous system.

Spindle Cells and Golgi Tendon Organs

Every muscle is full of kinesthetic receptors called *spindle cells* that detect changes in the muscle's length. These cells are like tiny gauges that tell your brain how long the muscle is at any given moment. Your brain continually uses this input to guide muscle movement.

Spindle cells are involved in a protective mechanism called the *stretch reflex.* As I mentioned in chapter 3, a reflex is an automatic muscular reaction that can be triggered by a variety of physical or emotional stimuli. When your doctor taps your knee with a rubber hammer, your leg muscles automatically react. The hammer tap causes the quadriceps muscle (on the front of the thigh) to contract rapidly, which triggers the muscle's stretch reflex, which causes your knee to jerk. When a muscle stretches too far and too quickly it is in danger of being torn. The spindle cells switch on a reflex that halts the lengthening of the muscle by strongly contracting it before it tears. If you fall asleep in a lecture hall or a theater and your head drops suddenly, then shoots back up, that is an example of the stretch reflex. The spindle cells in your neck muscles detect the dangerously rapid stretching of the muscles in the back of your neck, which triggers a reflexive contraction of those muscles and pulls your head back. This protective reaction prevents your neck muscles from being torn by an overly rapid stretch.

Tendons contain kinesthetic receptors, called *Golgi tendon organs*. These tendon organs continuously detect and send the brain information about the amount of tension and effort occurring within the tendon. Like spindle cells, Golgi tendon organs also have a protective reflex function, but the action is the opposite of the stretch reflex. In the Golgi reflex, when tension on a tendon exceeds a certain amount, the muscle automatically *releases,* preventing the tendons from being torn off the bone. This can be seen sometimes during arm wrestling competitions. When the contestants are evenly matched, there is a tremendous amount of tension on the tendons in the forearm. Occasionally, during one of these matches that appear to be a tie, the arm of one of the wrestlers will suddenly give out completely and be slammed onto the table by his opponent. In this case, the Golgi tendon organs triggered a reflex that caused the arm muscles to release instantly. Even though that caused the wrestler to lose the match, it saved him from ripping the tendons in his arm.

The spindles cells and tendon organs that initiate muscle reflexes also function as gauges for how long a muscle is allowed to be. The brain uses the kinesthetic information it receives to set these gauges, which prevent muscles from going beyond a certain length. Your degree of muscular tension is the result of how the gauges are set at any given moment.

Even though these gauges are controlled automatically by your nervous system in a feat of unimaginably complex coordination, you have the potential to override and change their settings at any moment. Have you ever seen a dancer drop his head suddenly as part of a specific dance move? Why isn't the same protective reflex activated in his neck muscles that would have been activated if he had fallen asleep in a lecture? Even if the head and neck movement is exactly the same in each case, the dancer's intention to drop his head instantaneously changes the muscle gauges so they fit the movement range he intends to perform. The muscle gauges are adaptable enough to change whenever the brain tells them to. The dancer's thoughts and desires can override the automatic settings of the gauges. This amazing system is at work all day long, allowing you to make movements whenever you wish and always returning the muscles to their baseline (default) length when the activity is finished.

Muscle Strength, Muscle Tone, and Relaxation

The physical health and performance fields tend to overemphasize the importance of muscle strength and ignore the importance of kinesthetic awareness. The pervasive yet questionable reliance on strength is evident in the way most health care professionals approach physical rehabilitation, in the way athletes and performers are trained, and in the way the commercial media shape popular culture. Health care professionals and athletic trainers tend to conclude that muscle weakness is the cause of any back pain, lack of athletic skill, or posture imbalance and that strengthening is the universal solution for every problem involving the muscles.

What exactly is muscle strength? Strength is a physical property of a muscle, referring to its size. At a microscopic level, muscles are largely made up of protein filaments arranged lengthwise along the muscle tissue. Strength is determined by the number of filaments within a muscle: the more filaments, the more physical force the muscle can exert. Imagine two people trying to push a car out of a snowbank. If three more people come to help them, the group of five will exert more force than the original two. Five people are stronger than two because they have more muscles to use. In the same way, a muscle with more filaments packed into it is a stronger muscle. When you lift weights for exercise, your muscles become stronger because the feeling of resistance from the weights sends a signal to your body to add more protein filaments into each exercised muscle. This is why weight lifters eat so much protein.

Although muscle strength is undoubtedly important, muscle tone is equally important. Technically, muscle tone is the tension in a muscle when you are at rest. It is the result of the muscle's relationship to the nervous system. Since the nervous system interconnects all parts of the mind, body, and emotions, muscle tone is a reflection of the whole person.

Muscle tone affects how muscles function and how much control you have over them. Lacking the kinesthetic awareness to use and relax your muscles efficiently reduces your ability to use their strength. Thus, the effective strength of your muscles depends in part on your kinesthetic awareness. Muscle strength is not useful if it is not coupled with muscle awareness.

Muscle tone can be rated along a continuum from low to high. People with low muscle tone tend to be slow to respond and sluggish, and people with high muscle tone tend to be quick to respond and jumpy. Healthy muscle tone is somewhere between the extremes, where a person has the capacity for both relaxation and quick responsiveness.

Muscle tone is always present in your body. The tension level of the tone may change from moment to moment, but it does not turn off. Muscle tone does not produce obvious movement; rather, it stabilizes your bones. For example, if you are sitting still on a bench, the muscle activity keeping you balanced is your muscle tone. If you are currently sitting up to read this book but are giving no thought to your posture, your muscle tone is automatically maintaining your upright position.

When you require muscle activity for movement beyond maintaining one position, your muscle tone is temporarily altered to move your bones as the activity requires. This is similar to how the protective muscular reflexes can be overridden, as in the earlier example of a dancer allowing his head to drop suddenly. Movement commands from your brain can temporarily increase muscle tone to make a movement happen. For example, a great deal of leg muscle movement is needed to make a jump shot in basketball. If you are standing still and holding a basketball, the muscle tone in your legs is allowing you to maintain your position without falling over. But this muscle activity, or tone, is not sufficient to make your legs move so you can jump. As you jump, the muscle tone in your legs increases temporarily, allowing the larger leg movements of jumping to occur. After the jump, when you are standing again, the muscle tone level will return to what it was before you jumped.

Your muscle tone can change if your emotional or mental state changes. Imagine that you are watching an enjoyable movie. Your shoulder muscles are fairly relaxed. Suddenly, a frightening scene causes your shoulder muscles to become tense. The tone (tension) of those muscles has become higher because of the emotion of fear. Conversely, when someone faints, there is such a rapid drop in muscle tone that the muscles become too relaxed to support the skeleton, and the person falls down.

In the context of muscle tone, *relaxation* is a relative term. When I use the term *relaxed,* I mean the right amount of tension. It means that your muscle tone is neither too high nor too low. Under ordinary conditions, your muscles are never absolutely relaxed. Your joints rely on the tension from your muscle tone to help hold your bones together, so completely relaxed muscles would put your joints at risk of dislocation. Interestingly, if you are under general anesthesia, the part of the brain that controls your muscle tone is deactivated and your muscles relax completely. In this state, your body must be moved with great care, because you lack the basic muscle tension required to protect your joints from injury or dislocation.

Relaxed muscles are not necessarily weak. Remember, the nervous system tells the muscles what to do and when to do it. Ideally, muscles would be able to respond fully to the directions they receive. The nervous system can access relaxed muscles better than tense muscles. This means that relaxed muscles can be used more fully than tense muscles, resulting in a feeling of greater strength.

To some extent, muscle strength and muscle tone overlap. In general, any physical activity causes muscle tone to increase. During physical activity, the neuromuscular system actively organizes muscle movement, and this movement increases tone. For this reason, any exercise that increases strength, such as weight training, tends to increase muscle tone as well. During periods of physical inactivity, the neuromuscular activity decreases, which results in a general decrease in both muscle tone and strength. For example, if a person remains in bed for six weeks due to illness, his leg muscles will become lower in tone, as well as weaker and smaller.

Muscle Contractions and Pain

The most common obstacle to proper muscle function is pain. Pain is the main reason that people consult me, either privately or in an exercise class. What exactly is pain? It is a sensation that occurs when the pain receptors at the ends of your sensory nerves are stimulated. In general, recurring muscular pain can be divided into two categories: neuromuscular pain and myofascial pain. Neuromuscular pain is the result of contracted muscles, while myofascial pain is caused by strain on the connective tissue. Most often, these two conditions occur simultaneously.

Neuromuscular Pain

A contracted muscle is one that does not disengage easily. It is really an involuntary muscular contraction, because you did not intentionally ask the muscle to engage and therefore cannot intentionally ask it to relax. A contracted muscle is constantly working and tense. A *muscle spasm* is a strong, painful, involuntary muscle contraction. When a muscle is in spasm, its tone is very high, and it is unable to return easily to its normal tone.

A muscle requires energy to do its job, just as a car engine requires gasoline. The energy that activates muscles comes from the food we eat and the air we breathe. A car engine produces waste by-products in the form of exhaust; muscles produce waste by-products in the form of a chemical called *lactic acid,* which causes the muscles to ache.

If your muscle tension comes from chronic muscle contractions, those tense muscles are constantly working and creating lactic acid. In this state, it is difficult for your circulatory system to remove the lactic acid from the muscle tissues. When lactic acid remains trapped in these tissues, it irritates the pain receptors in the muscles, sending a pain response to the brain. The result is constant pain. Tense muscles work harder and use up more energy than relaxed muscles. Therefore, they ache more and feel more fatigued than relaxed muscles.

Pain can also occur when muscles react to strain, pressure, or pain by contracting reflexively. This automatic reaction is known as the *pain reflex*. For instance, if you accidentally hit your thumb with a hammer, the pain in your thumb will cause your hand muscles to contract automatically. This natural response can become a problem when a muscle pain in one place (your thumb) triggers the pain reflex in another (the hand muscles). The reflexive muscle contraction ends up compounding the original pain because contracted muscles can become very tense, thus stimulating pain sensors that respond to pressure. This becomes a vicious pain cycle caused by a reaction to pain. Another example of this cycle can be seen when a person has whiplash, a condition in which the ligaments of the spine are injured, causing pain. As a result of this pain, the neck and upper back muscles will contract reflexively and violently. Contraction of these muscles compresses the neck even more, which causes more pain in the initial injury area.

Pain-causing muscle activity usually occurs below your level of awareness. For example, when you lie down at night to go to sleep, your muscles should relax, since you are not moving and have little need for muscle activity. No purpose is served by using energy to keep your muscles engaged while you are resting. In reality, however, many people find it difficult to let go of tension even when they rest, because they have lost the ability to control muscle relaxation.

A client will often tell me, "I have a tight muscle in my neck." More accurately, that client has a muscle that is *being tightened* in his or her neck. If you think of a muscle simply as an object that is tight, you might conclude that you have nothing to do with its behavior, as if it had a mind of its own. This faulty impression often gives rise to the feeling that you are a victim of circumstances beyond your control. In contrast, if you think of a muscle as something that is being tightened, the implication is that someone is tightening it. That someone is *you,* even if you are not aware of it and do not wish to do so. Muscles do not have minds of their own—they have your mind. Even though you have unconsciously trained your muscles to be tight, you can consciously retrain them to relax. If you become kinesthetically aware to the extent that you can sense what your body is doing, you can regain intentional control over your muscle behavior.

Myofascial Pain

Continuous muscle contractions can pull on the myofascial fabric with enough force to distort it. Over time, this fabric can become rigid, causing postural strain and restricting freedom of movement. This painful condition is sometimes referred to as *myofascial pain,* or *myofascial strain.*

Myofascial pain occurs when the compression of prolonged muscle tension or distorted posture causes the layers of myofascia to shorten and adhere to each other, resulting in restricted movement. It is not unlike a piece of plastic wrap that has become crinkled and stuck together in some places, so it is not as long and wide as it was originally. This can also occur when scar tissue forms after surgery or an injury. Scars are made of connective tissue. Myofascial restrictions such as these can be helped greatly by hands-on treatment, such as physical therapy, that manually releases the myofascial layers. Such treatments from a skilled practitioner can range from gentle to forceful, depending on the circumstances.

Most commonly, myofascial pain occurs in combination with neuromuscular pain. For example, if you have been experiencing hip pain and inflexibility for five years, the pain may be the result of myofascial shortening, but it may also be the result of muscle contractions caused by DMPs. People often believe that their tense and painful muscles are stuck together, because that's typically how they feel. However, that is frequently not the case. I have worked with countless people who felt their apparently "stuck" muscles let go in an instant as a result of gentle movement exercises that altered their kinesthetic awareness—with no prying apart or stretching of muscles involved. In these cases, their inflexibility clearly had more to do with a DMP than with actual fascial adhesions.

The neuromuscular and myofascial domains overlap, so it can be difficult to isolate their effects in practice. Fortunately, there is really no need to, as long as the therapeutic method is comprehensive. The muscular retraining exercises in this book address both neuromuscular and myofascial causes of pain. I have seen many clients make tremendous gains from simply doing these exercises. However, for multifaceted pain problems, people often require the helping hands of a skilled therapist to correct specific neuromuscular or myofascial issues. In these cases, the therapist uses hands-on procedures to return clients to a state where they can independently take over the work by using muscular retraining exercises.

Muscular Reactions to Injuries and Mishaps

Physical strain can be a cause of ongoing muscle contractions. If you experience this type of strain, you might assume you have hurt yourself, even if there is no clear evidence of an injury. But that may not be the case. *Injury* refers to an event where some structure in the body has been physically damaged. In contrast, a *muscular reaction* is a muscle contraction that does not involve any actual physical damage. Rather, it is a protective contraction in response to a strong sensory input, such as your arm being quickly pulled away from your shoulder joint or your back hitting the pavement after you've slipped on ice. An injury always has a corresponding muscular reaction, but a muscular reaction does not always have a corresponding injury.

Pain from Injuries: Stuart

When a musculoskeletal injury or strain occurs, an automatic protective reaction occurs in the nearby muscles. This reaction involves stretch reflexes and pain reflexes (discussed earlier in this chapter). For instance, if you accidentally step in a hole while running, your ankle might twist quickly. The instant this occurs, the stretch reflexes of the twisted muscles will trigger an intense contraction of those muscles. If the strain on your muscles is not too severe, the stretch reflexes may prevent your ankle from being injured. However, if the strain is too great, you may damage a ligament or break a bone. Whether you sustain an actual injury or not, any experience of pain triggers a pain reflex, which also causes intense muscle contractions. Automatic muscular contractions near an injury effectively immobilize the injured area, preventing painful movement. Moving an injured area tends to injure it further, since the tissues need to heal before they can be moved safely.

Your body is genetically programmed to heal itself. Sometimes healing occurs naturally; sometimes you need help in the form of a cast, a sling, or maybe even surgery. Bones are not the only structures that can be injured. Soft-tissue injuries, such as torn muscles and sprained ligaments, damage the more flexible structures in the body. Associated bruising and swelling indicate that cells, blood vessels, and connective tissues have been injured. Healing occurs when your body gradually clears out the debris from the injury and eventually repairs the injured tissues.

The protective stretch and pain reflexes from an injury can result in muscles that remain intensely contracted if the reflexes never turn off. This can happen when a long period of severe pain follows an injury. The pain and rigidity from such continuous muscle contractions can greatly impair movement, even after the injury has healed. I have seen many people who endure persistent pain long after a traumatic injury has been repaired. For example, workers who fall from high ladders or underneath scaffolding, pedestrians who are hit by a truck or car, and skiers who sustain multiple fractures in downhill accidents can suffer from impaired movement or pain after their injuries have healed.

One such person was fifty-year-old Stuart, who was injured while cutting down a huge tree. After severing a large limb, Stuart found himself in its path as it fell. The limb struck his leg, and he was thrown from the tree. His shattered right thigh bone was repaired by a skilled orthopedic surgeon, and in time, it was good as new. In spite of his medical good fortune, Stuart walked with a limp and had constant pain in his right thigh and hip for many months after the bone had healed. He did stretching and strengthening exercises for his leg and hip, but they did little to help.

When I first saw Stuart, he was using a cane. Although he had formerly been a long-distance runner, he was now only able to walk carefully for a few minutes on a treadmill before experiencing muscle spasms in his right thigh. He had muscle contractions that just wouldn't quit.

Without realizing it, Stuart's diligent efforts to strengthen and stretch his muscles had only made them contract more intensely. His muscle tension was the result of protective muscular reactions that would not turn off. His stretch reflexes were still actively trying to prevent his leg from being torn off his body—many months after the accident. With such intense stretch reflexes (remember, these are reflexes that prevent stretching) at work, his attempts to stretch the tight muscles simply triggered even stronger contractions. To make matters worse, his strengthening exercises, which involved forcefully engaging his leg muscles, encouraged the contracted muscles to remain contracted. In short, Stuart's strengthening and stretching exercises had reinforced his problem.

Using corrective movement exercises, hands-on manipulation, and alignment techniques, I helped Stuart to release the contracted muscles in his leg and to unlearn the habits he had developed by walking with a limp for six months. After five sessions and a fair amount of home exercise, Stuart was able to walk without pain. Two months later, Stuart was once again running on trails through the woods.

Pain from Muscular Reactions: Ted

Structural and soft-tissue injuries always hurt. But even if no injury occurs, the protective muscle contractions of the initial stretch reflexes can be painful. Although these reflexes may successfully minimize or even prevent an injury, the pain from the resulting muscle contractions can trigger pain reflexes, which in turn give rise to more contractions and more pain. In this way, a series of muscular reactions that give rise to pain after an event can masquerade as an actual injury. When you have an injury, you should treat it as an injury, and eventually it will heal. However, when you have pain from a muscular reaction and you mistakenly deal with it as if it were an injury, you will not succeed in turning off the muscular reaction. Healing an injury requires time and the proper medical treatment. Turning off a protective muscular reaction requires relaxation and retraining. An injury and a muscular reaction are two distinct situations. They are not mutually exclusive, but they are fundamentally different.

A personal experience showed me how easily a protective reaction can be mistaken for an injury. I was loading luggage into the backseat of my car during the aftermath of a big storm. As I turned to walk away from the car, a strong gust of wind blew the car door closed. My right arm was caught and forced backward by the closing door. I managed to pull my hand away just before the door slammed closed. I immediately felt a sharp pain in my right shoulder. The pain increased when I moved that shoulder.

I tried to continue loading luggage, but each time I tried to lift anything, I felt severe pain in my shoulder. The pain was so sharp that I thought I had seriously injured myself. I starting going over the possibilities of what might be wrong. Had I torn my shoulder muscles? Had I sprained the ligaments in my shoulder? Would I be able to manage everything on the trip I was about to take?

I decided to lie down and relax. When I focused my attention on my shoulder, I could feel that the muscles were all extremely tense. I rubbed the shoulder with my left hand, pressed a few sore muscle points near it, and consciously focused on relaxing the whole shoulder. After about fifteen minutes, I noticed that much of the pain was gone. I got up and found that I could lift the remainder of the luggage with only a little pain. I finished loading the car and started on my trip. After about an hour, I stopped feeling the shoulder pain and never felt it again.

So what had happened? At first, I felt certain that I must have injured my shoulder because of the force of the accident and the severity of the pain. But within an hour of the incident, the pain was gone, which indicated that nothing had really been injured. I had experienced effective and powerful protective muscular reflexes in my shoulder. These reflexes may have helped keep my arm in the shoulder socket. The pain I felt was due to the muscular contractions of these reflexes. By massaging and relaxing my muscles, I was able to stop the reactions. When the muscle contractions stopped, so did the pain.

What might have happened if I had not stopped to relax my arm? Imagine that I finished loading the luggage with my left arm and went on my way. Ideally, the muscular reaction would have relaxed later on its own. On the other hand, if the muscular reaction had persisted, my shoulder would have continued to hurt, and the pain reflexes would have continued to cause the muscles to contract. I could have become trapped in a vicious cycle of pain causing muscle tension and muscle tension causing pain. Such a cycle could have gone on for hours, days, weeks, months, or years.

Such was the case with Ted, who came to me for a consultation about the pain in his shoulder. The pain began after he moved a pile of firewood from one place to another. Eventually, he began throwing large pieces of wood. At one point, he felt a sharp twinge in his right shoulder. He ignored it and it seemed to go away, so he continued moving the wood, albeit a little more carefully. The next day, his shoulder hurt if he tried to lift his right arm higher than the shoulder. He figured that he had "pulled a muscle" while hurling wood.

Ted's shoulder pain never went away. He reasonably suspected that he had torn or pulled something in his shoulder, because after three months, he still could not lift his arm above shoulder height without feeling a sharp pain. Ted was well over six feet tall, and he had always had a lot of upper body strength. He could not understand why throwing wood, which wasn't that heavy, would cause such a problem.

I explained to Ted that even if he had injured his shoulder, his body would likely have healed it by now. At the very least, the damage should have been partially healed. Yet Ted said the pain had not changed since the day after the event. I suspected right away that he was dealing with a protective muscular reaction that would not turn off. He thought he had a torn rotator cuff, which is the set of deep shoulder muscles that rotate the arm and help keep it in the shoulder socket. A torn rotator cuff, which in serious cases requires surgery, was a possibility. Because I didn't have x-rays of Ted's shoulder, I suggested that we look at the muscular situation to see what could be done in that regard, instead of assuming that he had an injury.

I had Ted lie down on my treatment table. By moving his right arm gently and pressing my hand on specific shoulder muscles, I was able to demonstrate to him that his shoulder was being controlled and restrained by reflexive muscular reactions. After about thirty minutes, Ted had regained enough kinesthetic awareness to be able to disengage the muscular reactions and reach his right arm above his shoulder without pain.

Ted told me that his body had been feeling gradually more tense, inflexible, and achy over the past few years. He spent most of his days in front of a computer and didn't get much exercise. Chronic tension in his shoulder made him susceptible to the problems he encountered stacking his woodpile because his baseline muscle tone was already high. Pain from a muscular reaction is always more likely to affect a person who has tense muscles and kinesthetic dysfunction than a person who does not.

If Ted had done nothing to correct his shoulder pain, it would likely have continued indefinitely. Unless some new input was added to his neuromuscular system in the form of appropriate kinesthetic exercises or hands-on manipulation, the muscle contraction in his shoulder would have become permanent. As a result, he would have eventually developed myofascial strains and restrictions. At some point, he probably would have simply stopped attempting to raise his right arm above his shoulder and just learned to live with it. I have seen countless similar scenarios, where a person assumes that his or her pain is caused by arthritis or some other malady. This is a complete misunderstanding of the situation.

When you experience pain after strenuous activity or a mishap, it may be impossible to know whether or how much your body has been injured. In the final analysis, it didn't really matter whether Ted was actually injured or not, because the resolution of his problem would have been the same in either case. He needed to regain the full use of his arm by releasing the reflexive muscular reactions. When he did that, his pain disappeared and did not return.

Knowing whether an injury has or has not occurred is important because it affects the way you think about your condition. If you believe you have an injury when your pain is actually caused by a protective muscular reaction, you will not take effective action in solving your problem. For example, I worked with a woman who experienced hip pain that she thought came from a pulled muscle. I asked her when she pulled it, and she told me that the mishap had occurred more than a year before. I told her that if she had injured the muscle that long ago, her body would probably have healed by now. Ever since she had hurt her hip, she had carried the vague concept of an injured, defective muscle in her mind.

Her concept of a pulled muscle excluded the possibility that she could do something about the pain. She had been hoping that it might go away some day. She thought there was something wrong with her muscles, but there wasn't. They were doing exactly what her nervous system was telling them to do—contracting. Because she misunderstood the cause of her problem, she had been doing strengthening exercises, which had done nothing to help her situation. In fact, those exercises, which involved pushing against resistance, may have caused her muscles to contract even more. There is only one solution for pain from muscles that are in a prolonged, involuntary contraction: stop the muscles from contracting.

Here is a bit of advice: If you continue to experience pain for months after a painful event and your doctor can find no evidence of structural injury, be on the lookout for muscular reactions as a possible cause of your pain. Muscular reactions can be corrected. Increasing kinesthetic awareness can help you regain control of your muscles. Instead of concluding that your body is irreparably damaged, you can retrain your neuromuscular system to relax your muscles and increase your flexibility.

Compensatory Muscular Reactions

When muscular reactions refuse to subside on their own, other muscles sometimes contract. This is called *muscular compensation*. In fact, a person may have many such contractions. Why muscular compensation occurs is explained by Ronnie's case.

Compounding Muscular Reactions: Ronnie

Ronnie, a thirty-three-year-old woman, whose car was struck head-on as she waited to make a left turn, experienced compounding reflexive muscular reactions after her original whiplash-related neck pain. Shortly after the accident, she returned to work as a waitress and began physical therapy. She expected the neck pain to subside gradually. After many months, however, the pain had not improved. The frequent dull headaches she'd experienced since the accident had become a constant headache, which periodically became a three- to five-day migraine. In addition to neck pain, she now had pain across the back of her shoulders, in her upper arms, down her spine, across her lower back, and in the back of her hips.

Staying out of work was not a financial option for Ronnie, whose main concern was raising an active three-year-old boy. She had admirable determination and simply continued handling her responsibilities in spite of the compounding pain. The only way she could deal with the constant headache was to take pain medication, which was very expensive and made her feel dopey. After a year of this, Ronnie's physician referred her to me for treatment.

Ronnie's problem began from protective reflexes, muscle contractions that had been activated naturally by the impact and pain of the accident. She had the impression that pain was gradually spreading throughout her body. In reality, the reflexes triggered by the accident affected muscles throughout her whole body, and because these muscles were constantly engaged, the pain from the resulting muscle fatigue seemed to spread. In addition, the reflexes had made her spine inflexible. To compensate for this inflexibility, the muscles of her shoulders, arms, and hips had to work harder to move against the resistance of her tense spinal muscles. Gradually, this compensation caused even more tension in her spinal muscles. All of this muscle tension and pain made her use her whole body differently, resulting in a new DMP. These muscular habits could be seen when Ronnie walked, because her head, torso, and pelvis didn't rotate naturally as she moved. When she turned to reach for something, her entire upper body moved as if it were frozen in one piece. By the time I saw her, she had gotten so used to moving like a cement block that she was unaware of it. The strengthening exercises she had done in physical therapy had not helped her because they did not address the basic issue of her original protective reflex reactions to the accident, which were the cause of the constant muscle contractions throughout her body.

When I first felt the amount of tension in Ronnie's neck and back muscles, I was not surprised she had a constant headache. Ronnie was skeptical of my explanation of how muscular tension could cause such debilitating headaches. She figured that since she had been in an automobile accident, the whiplash must have affected something in her head. But her doctors had correctly assessed that there was no injury there. Ronnie was becoming anxious because nothing explained the cause of her headaches. Her anxiety about never being able to relieve this situation only compounded the tension she already had.

Because her case was so severe, Ronnie required many sessions of hands-on therapy, along with slowly paced retraining exercises. Stretching exercises only caused her muscles to tighten. Also, she was so sensitive to pain that the gentlest massage of the back of her shoulders could cause her many days of severe pain and a massive headache. Pain she experienced after a hands-on treatment would reactivate her protective muscular reflexes, and she would be back at square one. Although she typically tolerated pain well, her extreme sensitivity was typical of individuals who endure pain for a prolonged period of time.

Ronnie's kinesthetic awareness increased, and her muscles began to relax. She realized that the many different places where she felt pain were all part of one interconnected muscular reaction. She could feel that her pain was caused by habitual muscle tension. Her kinesthetic awareness let her relax the tension during her day-to-day activities. Through daily practice of corrective exercises, Ronnie gradually retrained her muscles and improved the skeletal alignment of her back and neck.

The migraine headaches, which had been caused by the constant pulling from contracted muscles in the back of her neck, began to subside. Eventually, even the constant dull headache disappeared completely. After nearly six months of weekly visits, Ronnie was able to go sledding with her son. In fact, she told me that she got on the sled face down and went down the hill headfirst! To top it off, she was not even sore the next day. Clearly, the Ronnie I first met had been only a shadow of her former self, and now she had regained her usual vitality and spirit.

Ronnie's problem is not at all unique. If she had not chanced on a health care provider (in this case, me) who engaged her kinesthetic awareness to address the neuromuscular roots of her pain, it is likely that the pain would have continued indefinitely. Ronnie was trapped in a pain cycle from which she was unable to escape until she used her kinesthetic awareness to erase the DMP by retraining her muscles.

If Ronnie had undergone this therapy immediately after her accident rather than a year later, she likely would have improved much more quickly. The year she lived with the pain only caused her to brace herself against it more and more, which caused further pain. Not only did she have to resolve her body's reaction to the accident, she also had to resolve her body's reaction to the year of pain following the accident. Added to the mix was the tremendous amount of emotional strain and uncertainty she went through in that year.

Ideally, muscular retraining should begin as soon as possible after an accident and after any potential structural injury has been ruled out or treated. Early muscular retraining can reverse the reflexive reactions to an injury before they escalate and compound.

EXPLORATION 4

Lie on your back with your knees bent and your feet flat on the floor. Place a hand on each side of your waist. Bend to the right so that the right side of your pelvis moves toward your right shoulder. Do this without increasing the arch in your lower back. Use your right hand to feel your muscles tightening as you bend, making the right side of your waist shorter. These are your side abdominal muscles, or oblique abdominals (see illustration 5.4 on page 88). At the same time, notice how the left side of your waist lengthens.

Next, reverse the movement and bend to the left. Notice how you can bend your whole torso by using your oblique abdominals. Continue bending slowly in this fashion, alternating right and left sides, until you can clearly feel these muscles shortening and lengthening on the sides of your waist. Side bending is a necessary part of pelvis, back, and shoulder movement.

5

Carriage, Alignment, and Posture

Don't fight forces, use them.
—*Buckminster Fuller*

THIS CHAPTER includes the fundamental information that I share with my clients on the subject of body carriage, alignment, and posture. These three elements are controlled by your muscle function and your kinesthetic awareness. Your muscles move your bones, and your bones are the solid support for your muscles.

Carriage is literally the way you *carry* your body. It is the dynamic process by which you support and present yourself as an embodied person. How you carry yourself reflects how you feel physically and emotionally, your energy level, and your kinesthetic awareness, as well as many other things. There is no specific body position for good carriage, because it is a process of continuous readjustment. By contrast, posture is the position in which you *hold* your body, either intentionally or unintentionally. We have all heard the phrases "good posture" and "bad posture." For the purposes of muscular retraining, I'd like to encourage you to think of posture as how you habitually hold your body: it is a static, or still, position. Finally, the word *alignment* refers to skeletal alignment, which is a technical term that describes how your bones are lined up in relation to each other.

Easy Movement in the Field of Gravity

Your body has the potential to allow you comfortable, easy movement with little or no pain. When your body, mind, and emotions are in a harmonious relationship, you function as a *whole self*. Your whole self organizes your carriage. When your carriage is good, your alignment is well organized. As a result, your body feels better and your movements are fluid and graceful.

To appreciate how this works, it is important that you not limit your concept of gravity. *Gravity* refers to the attraction that all particles in the universe have to one another. Without this attraction, the material world would disintegrate. Since the earth is so much bigger than you are, its attraction keeps you attached to it. Unless you strap yourself into a rocket ship or a space shuttle and travel thousands of miles out of our atmosphere, you cannot escape the power of the earth's attraction for your body.

Gravity plays a large role in the structures of living creatures. These structures have been shaped by the elements involved in each creature's existence. These elements are both internal (sensory/motor awareness) and external (the earth's gravity). Life on earth developed within the pervasive field of its gravity, and the structure of our musculoskeletal system was shaped accordingly. Your body structure works with gravity to allow you to stand upright and move. If your body structure had not developed to accommodate for the earth's gravity, you wouldn't be able to move.

In spite of this, many people consider gravity to be a major obstacle to standing upright. For example, traditional anatomy books often refer to the spinal extensor muscles that run vertically along either side of the spine as the "antigravity muscles" (see the shaded area of illustration 5.1). This name mistakenly suggests that standing must involve fighting against gravity. If your alignment is well organized, gravity will support you. If your alignment is not balanced, gravity will pull you down.

The exercises in this book reinforce better carriage and alignment by balancing muscle tone and increasing kinesthetic awareness. When

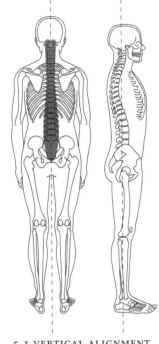

5.1 VERTICAL ALIGNMENT

you carry yourself well, you will be more centered. When your body alignment is sound, you will move easier and without pain.

Your Body's Tensegrity Structures

A simplified look at the musculoskeletal system will give you a picture of how it gives structural support to the body. The musculoskeletal system combines two different kinds of supportive structures: compressive and tensile. The *compressive* structures support the body because of their resistance to being compressed. The leg of a table is a compressive support because as the weight of the table presses down, the leg supports it by resisting the compression without being crushed. In your body, bones and cartilage are compressive supports that bear weight without being crushed.

The *tensile* elements of your musculoskeletal system provide support by resisting being stretched; they exert a pulling force. When you set up a tent, you can improve its stability by pulling the guy lines (the ropes attached to the outside of the tent) taut and staking them to the ground. The lines have a limit to how much they will stretch, and their tension is what stabilizes the tent walls. In your body, the muscles and ligaments are tensile supports that resist being stretched beyond a certain point.

Because your musculoskeletal system resists being compressed or stretched too much, the possibility exists for your body to hover somewhere between those two extremes. When it does, you can experience your body as being suspended from the inside. This internal suspension is described very well by the concept of tensegrity. The American physicist Buckminster Fuller created the term *tensegrity* by combining the words *tension* and *integrity*. According to Fuller's concept, the entire natural world is a construction that combines less flexible compression material with more flexible tensile material. His geodesic dome is an example of a tensegrity structure.

Consider a rock wall and a suspension bridge. The rocks in the lower part of the wall support the compressive forces of the rocks above them. The strength of the rocks determines how much weight can be loaded on top of the wall before the rocks at the bottom are crushed. The rock wall contains no tensile elements (except for bonding forces at the molecular level) to distribute the weight evenly. A suspension bridge, in contrast, uses cables to create a tensile (pulling) force that resists being stretched by the weight of the bridge, distributing that weight strategically through its supports.

Nature is full of three-dimensional structures that represent configurations of compression and tensile forces. In a natural tensegrity structure, the compression and tensile forces are distributed evenly, so the structure is supported from inside itself. The tensile components are arranged in such a way that the compression components can bear the maximum possible load using the minimum amount of energy. As a result, a tensegrity structure as a whole is stronger than its individual parts.

I have given you this brief description because your body is also a tensegrity structure. The weight of your body, which is supported by your bones, can be minimized by the efficient use of the tensile supports of your muscles and connective tissue (see chapter 4 for a discussion of fascia, ligaments, and tendons). When these compressive and tensile forces are in harmony, your body is expansive, balanced, and not bothered by gravity.

When you are standing, the weight of your body exerts a compressive force on your bones. This force is limited by the restraining tension of the fascia, which acts like shrink-wrap and is reinforced by muscles and ligaments. The fascia is loosely analogous to a web. Imagine a superstrong spiderweb suspended between two branches of a tree. Now imagine dropping a number of small twigs into the web so they are not touching one another. The twigs are analogous to bones. If you push and pull on one of the twigs, the entire web will conform to the force you exert. But the other twigs in the web (if they are strategically placed) will actually help the web maintain its general shape, because they resist being compressed. Between the tensile strength of the web and the compressive strength of the twigs, the structure of our imagined spiderweb will tend to keep the integrity of its shape and return to its original shape when the compressive forces cease.

Your body's remarkable tensegrity is such that the more your bones are moved in any given direction, the more strongly the connective tissues restrain them from moving too far. Your internal, three-dimensional web of connective tissue helps to suspend your bones.

The structure of a balloon provides another analogy to the tensegrity structure of your body. In a filled balloon, the forces of expansion and contraction are in harmony. The balloon's collapse is prevented by the support of the air inside, while the expansion is limited by the rubber around the outside. The balloon is in a state of suspension. The tensegrity does not depend on the balloon being right side up, upside down, or in any other position.

Like a balloon, your body does not depend on any particular position for its tensegrity. You can be standing, crawling, or walking on your hands. Tensegrity is the internal suspension built into the structure of your body, regardless of its position. The connective tissue supports the bones, while the bones support the connective tissue.

Your body is efficiently suspended from within. How you carry your-self is a result of how suspended you let yourself be.

Tensegrity for Internal Suspension

The idea of the body being suspended from within (tensegrity) can be very helpful for people who wish to have good carriage. Dancers, martial artists, circus performers, athletes, and others who carry them-selves with precision and balance are often aware of a sensation of suspension in their bodies and know how to maintain it. A mime artist climbing an imaginary ladder can give the impression of being suspended. A ballerina who balances on the point of one foot also conveys that impression. A tai chi master can be so suspended that he appears to be floating in the air.

We are born with an inherent ability to feel and use the internal suspension of our bodies. Take some time to observe the carriage and movement of young children. Toddlers often appear to be hov-ering, as if suspended from invisible strings. If you squeeze a child's legs while she is standing, you will feel that the muscles are rather re-laxed. She is using the minimum amount of muscular effort and max-imizing the use of her bones. Also, notice how a young child's head is balanced on top of the spine. The head is large and heavy, yet she manages to keep her head up with very little effort. Children naturally use their body's innate capacity for suspension to the maximum.

As a child grows, his movement learning is influenced by the move-ment of his parents, as well as by limits on his freedom of movement, such as excessive sitting (or slouching) in chairs and abridged free playtime. Emotional reactions that eventually become habitual will become rigid body postures. Because of all these troubling influences, a child's sense of internal suspension can eventually disappear, result-ing in poor carriage and alignment.

In light of your body's capacity to be suspended internally, it is limiting to think of your skeleton as merely a bunch of bones stacked on top of one another. The compressive supports of your bones are designed to work in conjunction with the tensile supports of your muscles. However, when your muscles are too tense or too slack, your bones lose their good alignment and their mechanical advantage for bearing weight. This overcompresses your joints and distends your ligaments and tendons, potentially damaging them.

Your muscles are the key to changing your carriage and improving your alignment. Your muscle tone determines how you carry yourself and how your bones are lined up in relation to each other. As you read in chapter 4, muscle tone can be constant, but it can also vary from one moment to the next. When muscle tone is balanced, not too tense and not too lax, the compressive and tensile supports work in concert, creating a feeling of internal suspension.

Muscle tone is influenced by your nervous system, your kinesthesia, your moods, and your self-awareness. Therefore, anything that affects the nervous system can affect muscle tone, including emotions, thoughts, diet, and lifestyle habits. You can change your muscle tone through exercise and awareness, which in turn improves your carriage and alignment. The more you are able to feel your internal suspension, the more flexible your movement will become and the less muscular pain you will have.

When your musculoskeletal system is suspended, its parts are not overly compressed. The bones don't grind against each other; the tendons and ligaments aren't injured by being under constant tensile strain. Movement feels more like an expansion than a contraction, and there is a minimum of friction. Less friction means that the individual parts require less energy to move. As a result, you save energy. Your movement feels easier, because it *is* easier.

Your Body's Balance Point

As I mentioned earlier, carriage is a process, not a rigidly held position. You can't maintain good carriage by holding a fixed position that produces unnecessary tension. Your neuromuscular system is flexible and fluid in nature. When your carriage is good, you can feel yourself moving, even when you appear to be standing still. Whenever you breathe, you are moving. Your nervous system continuously monitors the tiny movements of your bones and allows your muscles to release and take in slack wherever and whenever needed.

Rather than grabbing on to your bones and holding them in a fixed place, your muscles continually juggle them and allow them to balance properly.

When your bones are balanced in relation to each other, you are in good alignment. Ideally, when you stand up, your bones are hovering next to one another in such a way that the minimum amount of muscular energy is required to maintain their alignment. The better your alignment, the less muscular effort is required. Unnecessary muscular effort requires energy, which will ultimately result in muscle tension and pain.

The following simple exercise can help you get a feeling for how your bones can balance. Find some kind of pole or stick about three to five feet long, such as a yardstick, a broomstick, or a long dowel. Stand with the palm of one hand facing up, and balance the stick vertically on your palm. To keep the stick on end, you need to move your hand and arm. The more skilled you are at keeping the stick upright, the fewer arm and hand movements you need to use. You may notice that the stick seems suspended momentarily whenever it passes through its balance point. You cannot keep the stick fixed at the balance point, but you can keep it within a close range.

Like the stick, your bones have a balance point, and you have the ability to keep them within close range of it. For example, at the knee joint, the thighbone (femur) balances on top of the shinbone (tibia). While you are standing, attempt to balance your thighs on top of your calves. People often tell me that their legs feel unstable when they first do this. Their usual sense of stability comes from the immobility of locking their knees in a hyperextended position, so they are leaning back on their knee ligaments. When your upper leg is balanced on top of your lower leg, your knees will be neither locked backward nor bent forward, but somewhere in the middle. They will feel loose, which means they are free to move easily in any direction. Balance and security in your body comes from being comfortable with freedom of movement, not from holding yourself still or collapsing onto your ligaments.

Your body's balance point, or center of gravity, lies near the middle of your body, a little below your navel. In the physical science of mechanics, *center of gravity* refers to the location within an object around which its weight is balanced. Imagine that you are pushing against a large barrel, which is standing upright. If you push against the barrel below its center of gravity, the barrel will slide along the ground. If you push above its center of gravity, it will tip over. The barrel's exact center of gravity lies somewhere between these two extremes. I will refer to the general vicinity of your body's center of gravity as your body center.

The body center is sometimes referred to by the Japanese word *hara*, meaning "abdomen." For example, in the Japanese martial art of aikido, *hara* refers to the origin of movement as well as the physical center of movement. *Hara* is a useful term because it refers not only to the center of the body, but to the center of the whole person. In this book, the phrase "body center" has the same meaning as *hara*.

For the most part, the largest muscles in the body are closest to the body center, and the muscles become gradually smaller toward the extremities (legs, arms, and neck). The large muscles help maintain balance for the entire body by responding when any movement is made. For example, if you swing your arm in a large circle while standing, the muscles of your body center engage to help support your balance and assist the movement of your shoulder. The lumbar spine and pelvis are near the body center, so their alignment affects the balance of the entire body. The fundamental job of the muscles of the body center is to maintain the alignment of the pelvis and lumbar spine. When the pelvis and lumbar spine are misaligned, less central muscles must overwork for your whole body to be balanced. This can be the cause of constant muscle tension in the hips, legs, upper back, shoulders, arms, and/or neck.

Whole Movement

Because of the interdependency of the different parts of the body, a dysfunction in one part can cause trouble in another part. Here is an example: the lower back can be the ultimate source of wrist pain. How is that possible? Maybe you have tendonitis in your wrist because constant muscle strain in your arm is irritating your tendons. The constant muscle strain comes from moving your arm against the resistance of your inflexible shoulder. Your shoulder joint is inflexible because the shoulder blade (scapula) is misaligned. The scapula is misaligned because your upper spine is curved too much and your shoulder muscles are too tense. Your upper spine is curved too much because it is compensating for your unsupported lumbar spine, which has collapsed into a slumping posture (more on this later). Your lumbar spine has collapsed because your abdominal muscle tone is too low and your chronically tight hip muscles prevent your pelvis from maintaining balanced alignment. Thus, in a slow chain reaction, poor muscle tone and misalignment of the body center can result in wrist pain, or pain in any of the extremities. Poor alignment, muscular reactions from injury, and kinesthetic dysfunction—the usual culprits—interfere with easy movement.

There are more than two hundred muscles in the human body; none of them works alone. Even though you have the capacity to intentionally isolate and engage specific muscles, which can be a helpful therapeutic technique, you do not naturally move one muscle at a time or even one muscle group at a time. With every moment, your brain organizes your muscles in relation to the entire gestalt of your movement. This is the only way you can accomplish any kind of functional movement. Notice how many of your muscles you can feel working when you get up from a chair. If you only used one muscle at a time or only your leg muscles or back muscles, you would never be able to stand up.

When your carriage is internally suspended, every part of your musculoskeletal system works together evenly. You enjoy the distinct sensation of your movements requiring minimal effort, and the effort for any movement is spread throughout your entire body. This is tensegrity in action. Even ordinary movements, such as bending and walking, give rise to sensations of moving as a whole.

The simple action of throwing a ball can demonstrate the benefits of using your entire body. Throw a ball (or a small scarf, if you are inside) while keeping your body perfectly still, except for your throwing arm. Notice how the movement feels. You need to physically restrain the rest of your body to keep it still while you use your arm to throw. By restraining the rest of your body, you ultimately restrain your arm. This is how ongoing muscle tension in the back and shoulders affects the use of the arms. You might also notice that your movement feels distinctly robotic. If you always used your arm this way, you would eventually feel strain somewhere, because your arm would be working against your body's resistance every time it moved. Now throw the ball or scarf again, this time allowing your body to move along with your throwing arm. Notice how the movements of your legs and torso affect the use of your arm. The more your whole body works with your arm, the less work your arm needs to do. This is true of any movement you make: the more your whole body works together, the less any one particular area is strained, even if you use it repeatedly.

Another distinction can be made about whole movement. We are taught in anatomy class that muscles make bones move by contracting. From the perspective of muscle physiology, this makes sense, because it implies a locking up in order to move. From a whole-movement perspective, though, movement happens as the result of *releasing* muscles, not compressing them. Try this: Begin to walk forward from a standing position, and notice how much muscle effort you use to take a few steps. Now try again, but this time keep your muscles relaxed and imagine that your whole body is expanding in all directions. With that feeling, release your limbs as you walk. Notice how you are able to step forward with much less effort.

Alignment and Misalignment

The body as a whole maintains the curve, length, and flexibility of the spine. If your muscles hold your spine in a rigid posture, alignment problems will result. A well-supported and aligned spine is more like a curvy string of pearls than a straight column. The spine continually adjusts its position in response to the continual motion of your breathing. When your muscle tone is in balance, your spine can be flexible and strong at the same time.

This section covers the basics of skeletal alignment and how this alignment can go awry. First, we take a look at the natural shape of the spine, which is the basis for the alignment of the rest of the body.

Spinal Curvature

Living structures are rarely linear. More often, they are rounded, wavy, or spiral in shape. For example, the fibers within bones are curved, plants reach out toward the sun by curving their stems or branches, and DNA is shaped in a spiral. Even water moves in a curvy, spiral pattern, creating the serpentine shape of many rivers. Your spine, which is curved, is part of this great nonlinear natural heritage (illustration 5.2).

When a child is born, his spine is a C-shaped curve because he has been curled up in the fetal position. As the infant begins to lie on the ground, kick, reach, and look around, muscle tone develops in his torso, which changes his spine's concave curve to a shape that alternates between concave and convex. The lower back and neck curves become convex (when viewed from the front), while the curves of

5.2 SPINE

the tailbone and the chest remain concave. It is essential that infants spend time on the ground, facing the challenge of movement. This challenge is necessary for muscle development that produces healthy spinal curves. When infants are propped up in chairs before their spine is developed enough to support itself, they slump over in a position that interferes with good breathing. This initiates a movement pattern of collapsing the spine.

The spine and skull form a protective housing for the nerves of your central nervous system. In addition, the spine provides structural support for your body so that you can move and breathe in an upright position. It is not straight like a pole, but curved like a wave. The wavy spinal shape allows the spine to be both maximally movable and maximally stable. The strength of the spine is in its curves. Its wavy shape makes it resilient when it is compressed, like a spring.

The ideal shape of the lumbar curve is to be as long and as rounded as possible. It is a long, gradual arc. A good lumbar curve does not remain stuck in a rigid "correct" shape. The everyday movements of walking, bending, reaching, and so forth all require that the lumbar curve adjust to whatever movement is happening in the moment. It has a wave shape that can bend this way and that without losing its inner strength. The ability of the lumbar spine to be flexible yet maintain its long, gradual arc depends on the tone of the muscles that surround it.

The Psoas Muscle

The muscles that have the greatest influence on the function of the lumbar curve are the *psoas* (pronounced "so-as") *muscles* (illustration 5.3). These muscles (there is one on the left and one on the right) are attached to the front of the entire lumbar spine and the front of the pelvis. From the lumbar spine, they travel diagonally down and forward, over the front of the pelvis, attaching to the top of the insides of the thighs. The psoas muscles are perfectly situated to maintain the natural lumbar curve by encouraging the lumbar spine to bow forward. This will only happen if the psoas muscles have good muscle tone.

When psoas muscle tone is good, the lower back feels strong and stable, and the waist feels long. The majority of people I see with lower back and hip problems have poor muscle tone, and usually

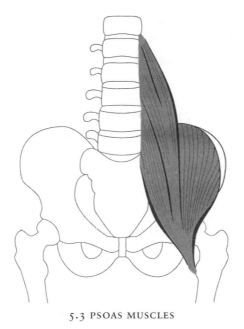

5.3 PSOAS MUSCLES

too much tension, in one or both psoas muscles. As a result, the psoas will not release or respond properly when needed. If a psoas is not released, it exerts a constant pull and strain somewhere in the hip or lower back. Also, it pulls on the spine in such way that can excessively flatten or exaggerate the lumbar curve. Psoas muscle strain can be relieved temporarily by lying on your back with your knees up and bent, and your lower legs supported by a low table or chair. Many people with lower back pain discover this position in their trial-and-error attempts to get comfortable.

Other Abdominal Area Muscles

The muscle tone of the abdominal wall also plays a crucial role in supporting the lumbar spine (illustration 5.4). If abdominal muscle tone is too tense, the rigidity of the abdominal wall interferes with your ability to breathe freely. If the muscle tone, particularly of the transverse abdominal muscle, is too loose, then the lumbar spine can shorten into a collapsed posture. The transverse abdominal muscles, which run horizontally, and the oblique abdominal muscles, which run diagonally, support the lumbar curve from the front and sides of the waist.

How much abdominal muscle tone do you really need? You may have noticed that young children are able to stand without a problem, yet they usually do not have highly developed abdominal strength. You do not need rock-hard abs to have good alignment. You need enough abdominal muscle tone to make your waist, which is the area between your pelvis and your ribs (front, back, and sides), as long as possible, *without* interfering with your breathing. A long waist is the key to a strong lower back and good alignment in the whole body. Several exercises in this book are specifically for this purpose.

Speaking of breathing, the lumbar curve also has an effect on your breathing. The primary breathing muscle is the diaphragm (see chapter 3). The diaphragm is a slightly dome-shaped muscle that connects the lower ribs to the lumbar spine, and its movement continuously changes the space inside your breathing cavity. When the

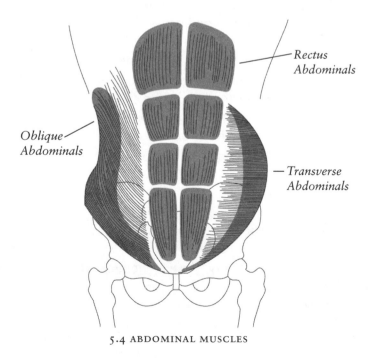

5.4 ABDOMINAL MUSCLES

diaphragm moves down, there is more space around the lungs and inhalation occurs. When the diaphragm moves up, there is less space around the lungs and exhalation occurs. Since the diaphragm is anchored to the lumbar spine, its function relies on the arc of the spine. Some people can feel a wavelike motion in their spine as they breathe, which is the natural effect that breathing has on a spine with a good lumbar curve and reasonably relaxed back muscles.

Lumbar Curve Distortions

As mentioned earlier, the ideal shape of your lumbar curve is as round and long as possible. If it is too round, then it becomes too short. If it is too long, then it becomes too straight. Any section of the spine can be distorted in three basic ways: curved laterally (sideways), exaggerated, or flattened.

LATERAL CURVE

A lateral curve is when the spine curves either to the left or to the right and is sometimes called *scoliosis*. There are two types of scoliosis. One usually develops in adolescence, when the growing spine becomes fixed in a lateral curve or in two opposing lateral curves. The cause of adolescent-onset scoliosis is unknown, but a dysfunctional psoas muscle is one of the likely factors. This type of scoliosis can cause pain problems later in life, because the spine becomes locked into its asymmetric position. With determination, the pain from this type of scoliosis can be mitigated by exercises that balance the muscles of the torso and legs and by awareness of alignment and body use. However, the underlying structural lateral curve of the spine remains.

The other type of scoliosis is a lateral spinal curvature caused by alignment issues other than the development of the spine itself. This is sometimes referred to as functional scoliosis. There are many possible causes of this, including back injury. A leg injury that causes a person to use one leg differently from the other and that causes the pelvis to tilt to one side is another common cause of a lateral spinal curve. In my experience, functional scoliosis usually involves a severely contracted psoas muscle on one side of the body. The psoas contraction causes that entire side of the waist and hip to compress. Other abdominal and back muscle contractions become involved as well. The result is that the lumbar spine shortens (becomes concave) on that side.

One way to see functional scoliosis in a person is to compare the length of the left and right side of the waist. For example, if the right side of the waist is shorter, then the spine will be concave on the right, as if the torso is always bending a bit to that side. Since functional scoliosis is not a structural problem with the spine itself, it can be greatly reduced with exercise and alignment improvement. Of course, years of uneven strain can negatively affect the joints and discs of the spine. Nonetheless, evening out the muscle tone on both sides of the spine and regaining kinesthetic awareness of body symmetry can bring the spine into balance.

EXAGGERATED LUMBAR CURVE

When a psoas muscle is too tense, it can cause the lumbar curve to become exaggerated, so that the top of the pelvis is tipped forward. In some cases, this psoas tension will cause lower back pain.

Another common problem is when the psoas does not support the lumbar spine, either because muscle tone is low or because the muscle is involuntarily contracted. When the lumbar spine is not supported by the psoas, the muscles that run vertically down both sides of the back of your spine take over and overwork themselves. These muscles are collectively called *spinal extensors* (illustration 5.1), and they span short and long distances from the head to the tailbone. If the spinal extensor muscles are habitually contracted because the psoas is not doing its job, you will probably have an exaggerated lumbar curve. In fact, all of your back muscles will be shortened so that your spine as a whole is bent backward (like an archer's bow). This does not allow your body weight to balance easily through your spine and pelvis. To deal with this disadvantage, the spinal extensors contract even more to help you maintain your balance. These muscle contractions are another possible cause of back pain.

Conventional wisdom states that the spinal extensor muscles need to be strong to maintain the natural curves of the spine, as well as to keep you in an upright position. I rarely encounter a person with significant weakness in these muscles. The real problem is often that one or both psoas muscles are not supporting the spine, causing the spinal extensors to become tense. The spinal extensors appear to have a weakness problem because their chronic tension causes kinesthetic dysfunction (see chapter 2).

People often tell me that they have been taught in an exercise class to decrease their lumbar curve by "tucking" their pelvis. They demonstrate this tucking by tightening the abdominal and buttock muscles. As mentioned earlier, the tone of the transverse abdominals plays a key role in supporting the lumbar spine. However, using the rectus abdominals to forcefully hold your pelvis in a fixed position is not a good idea because the front of your waist becomes shortened. Also, there is no need to tighten the buttocks. All of this effort to tuck the pelvis can make the lower back and hips inflexible and possibly even flatten the natural lumbar curve. The way to correct an exaggerated lumbar curve is to relax the back muscles and support the spine with the psoas and transverse and oblique abdominals.

FLATTENED LUMBAR CURVE

When the lumbar curve is flattened, it loses the benefit of its innate shape. Instead of acting like a spring that bounces under the weight of the body, the spine becomes more like a rod that is being driven straight down with every step. Also, the flattened lumbar curve seriously compresses the spinal discs, which over time causes them to tear, break, or deteriorate.

The lumbar curve becomes flattened when the abdominal area becomes compressed. Three common causes for this are years of a slouching sitting posture, abdominal muscle contractions following surgery, and abdominal and psoas muscle contractions caused by fear. In the first case, the slouching sitting posture involves psoas muscles that are not actively maintaining the spinal curve while the person is sitting, so the pelvis rolls backward and the lumbar curve becomes concave (from the front). In the other two cases, the lumbar curve is flattened because the tightened rectus abdominal and/or psoas muscles are crunching the waist.

Some people do not appear to have an overtly flattened lumbar curve when they are standing, yet when they bend at the hips, such as in reaching down to pick up something on the ground, their lumbar curve is flattened by the pull of their tight hip muscles. This condition is very common, even in people who appear to have a pronounced lumbar curve when standing up. The condition of the hip muscles has considerable bearing on the lumbar spine. The result of a lifetime of bending and sitting with tight hip muscles can be a flattened lumbar spine.

Collapsed Posture

If you observe your fellow human beings, you can see many who are stuck in a set posture of one type or another. The habitual posture a person holds might be a reflection of his or her kinesthetic awareness, occupation, emotional life, history of injuries, genetics, and overall self-awareness. A person with a balanced carriage has good alignment from head to toe (illustration 5.5). In my experience, the most commonly held posture is what I call *collapsed posture* (illustration 5.6). It is most easily recognized in the middle of the body, where the weight of the upper body shortens the waist and compresses the lumbar spine. A person with collapsed posture has kinesthetic dysfunction in the waist muscles (if not elsewhere). It is as if he has abandoned the support of his body. The spinal curves become compressed and distorted due to the lack of muscular support and balance, while many of the other muscles compensate by tightening up.

A person with collapsed posture often appears tired. I suspect that spending much of our time in chairs has contributed to the preponderance of this malady, because chairs allow us to abandon much of our muscle tone without falling over. The chair holds you up, so your muscles can take a vacation. I don't think chairs are the only cause, however. The collapsed posture reflects a lack of vital energy and a lack of tone in the body center. Since it is so common, I suspect it has much to do with general lifestyle.

Because the body moves and functions as a whole, collapsed posture affects not only the spine, but the whole body. The collapse can be seen as beginning at the waist when the tone of the psoas and abdominal muscles do not support the lumbar spine sufficiently. This causes the natural long arc of the lumbar spine to collapse from the

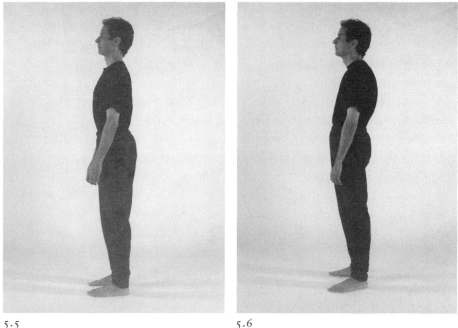

5.5   5.6

weight of the upper body pressing down on it, compressing the lumbar vertebrae, discs, and joints. Depending on which way the pelvis is tilted, this collapse of the waist muscles can cause the lumbar curve to be either flattened or exaggerated. For example, sitting back in a soft couch tends to collapse the waist by flattening the lumbar curve because the shape of the couch encourages the rim of the pelvis to tilt back. On the other hand, many people with a collapsed standing posture are actually exaggerating their lumbar curve by locking their knees and pushing their pelvis forward. Standing this way makes the lower back appear shorter, like a spring that is being compressed.

In the standing collapsed posture, the pelvis is often too far forward. To maintain overall balance, the chest and upper back are too far backward. Because of this, the naturally concave thoracic spine—the twelve vertebrae to which the ribs attach on each side—caves in even more, the shoulders round forward, and the upper chest narrows.

Since the weight of the chest is too far back, the head must be positioned far forward to prevent the person from falling over backward. This puts the neck in a diagonally forward position. Since the neck is slanted, the head looks down. In order to look straight ahead, the head must tilt back, which is done by tensing up and shortening the back of the neck. As a result, the neck takes on a collapse similar to the one in the lumbar spine.

Not surprisingly, many people with collapsed posture have chronic neck pain. The neck can easily bear the weight of a ten-pound head if the head is balanced on top of the spine, but the neck muscles will always be tense if the head is too far forward. Attempting to correct this by pulling the head back does not help, because the rest of the body's alignment is still collapsed, which is the cause of the forward head position in the first place. The head soon finds itself in front of the torso again, which prevents the whole body from falling over backward. To change the carriage of the head, along with the associated neck misalignment and pain, the alignment of the entire spine needs to change.

Pelvic Tilt

The *pelvis* is the configuration of bones that connects the spine to the legs. The left and right sides of the pelvis are connected in front via the *pubic bone*. In back, they are connected to the *sacrum,* which is the base of the spine. The pelvis can function and move as an entire unit, but the left and right sides are also capable of small but significant independent movements. At the base of the pelvis are two rocker-shaped bones known as the *sit bones*. If you sit upright on a hard bench or chair, you can feel your sit bones pressing into the chair.

The top of the pelvis can be level, tilted forward, or tilted backward. Because the pelvis connects to the spine, its position affects the curve of the lumbar spine. When the pelvis is level, the lumbar spine has its natural curve. When the pelvis is tipped forward, the lumbar curve increases, and when the pelvis is tipped backward, the lumbar curve flattens.

The pelvis can also be tilted from side to side (laterally), so that one side is higher than the other. This remarkably common situation causes more compression on one side of the waist than the other (the reversible type of scoliosis mentioned earlier). Since the pelvis is connected to the base of the spine, the spine must compensate for the lateral tilt by curving sideways. You can see this kind of lateral tilt if you place a brick under the base of a houseplant, so the whole pot is tilted diagonally. As the plant grows, its top eventually straightens out. However, the base of the plant remains bent, because the pot is still tilted. Often, a person with a laterally tilted pelvis does not have a tilted head. Like the base of the tilted houseplant's stem, some part of the spine has had to curve sideways to keep the head in a level position.

Many muscles connect the bones of the pelvis, spine, and legs. A lateral pelvic tilt can result when the psoas and other hip, waist, and leg muscles contract and shorten on one side of the body in a different way than on the other side. This kind of imbalance commonly occurs after an injury to some part of one leg or foot. In this case, the muscles automatically pull or twist the pelvis to one side or the other, either as a response to pain or to help the individual walk with an injury, such as a sprained ankle. Tilting the pelvis laterally will take some weight off the painful or injured leg.

A pelvis that is tilted laterally can give you the impression that one of your legs is shorter than the other, because that is how it feels when you stand and walk. If your left and right leg bones actually differ in length, your pelvis will tilt toward the shorter leg. In my experience, an actual difference between bone lengths is unusual, but the *appearance* of a difference in leg length is very common. Usually, apparent differences in leg length are due to muscle contractions of the psoas and other hip and waist muscles that pull the leg too far up toward the pelvis and tilt the pelvis laterally.

To help you picture this lateral pelvic tilt, imagine a puppet or a flexible doll that is hanging by its head so that its feet lightly touch the floor. Now imagine that its pelvis is titled laterally, so that one side of the waist is shorter than the other. The leg on the shorter side will lift off the floor. If the puppet suddenly came to life and attempted to walk in this position, it would have the feeling that one leg was shorter than the other and possibly even walk with a limp. The puppet has an apparent leg length difference, not an actual leg length difference. The problem is not in the legs, but in the waist and pelvis.

Pelvic Rotation

The pelvis can also be rotated laterally, meaning that the front of one side is farther forward than the front of the other side. In a standing position, place your hands on the left and right front of your pelvis to feel if one side is farther forward than the other. Or lie face down on the floor. Does it feel like one side of your pelvis is pressing into the floor more than the other side? If so, it means that your pelvis is rotated. This rotation is a misalignment again caused by muscle contractions in the psoas and other hip, waist, and leg muscles.

The *sacroiliac joints*—the joints between the left and right sides of the pelvis and the sacrum—can become painful when the pelvis is rotated in this way. Pain from either of these joints is felt in the back of the pelvis, to the right or the left of center. Although little motion is possible at the sacroiliac joints, the motion is essential to body movement. Misalignment of the pelvic bones can compress the sacroiliac joint and cause pain. As with other problems of skeletal misalignment, the muscles need to be retrained to correct the problem for the long term. In this case, the muscle tone of the psoas, abdominal, hip, and thigh muscles need to be corrected.

Movement at the Hips

Remember that the hip is the joint where the ball-shaped top of the thighbone connects to the cup-shaped socket of the pelvis. This extremely strong joint is able to bend like a hinge and rotate like a ball. If you observe toddlers playing, you will notice that they bend at their hips when they want to get closer to the ground. If they continue bending the hip joints, they eventually end up squatting. Squatting with both feet flat on the floor is a natural position, as evidenced by the fact that small children can do it so easily. In cultures where people live without chairs, squatting for long periods of time is common for people of all ages.

The ability to bend at the hips is a critical function, because it allows you to bend down without distorting the natural length of your spine. I have worked with many people who had hip muscles so inflexible that they were unable to move the hip joint without pain. Often, these people could not remember the feeling of bending at the hips, so they bent at the waist instead. This is kinesthetic dysfunction. When this happens, I show the person exactly where the hips are and how they bend. Most of these people do not realize that the hip joint is as low as it is, on the same level as the pubic bone. If you push your fingers firmly into the front of the hip joints as you bend, you will notice that you can indeed bend at your hips rather than your waist. This understanding may help to initiate the process of regaining important kinesthetic awareness.

Pay attention to how you bend down when you are washing your hands at a sink. How do you get your body low enough to reach the water? Does your spine become concave, because you are making a hinge out of your waist? Or do you bend your hips, knees, and ankles while keeping your waist long? Try keeping your spine long and bending your hips, knees, and ankles the next time you wash your hands. If this feels awkward, it means that you habitually bend at the waist and do not fully use your leg joints.

Remember, one function of your hip, knee, and ankle joints is to allow you to raise and lower your body without crumpling your spine. The nerves and blood vessels of the spine function best when they have plenty of space, not when they are squished and pinched. To keep your spine long, you need to use your hip joints fully. Many of the exercises in this book will help with this. Until you progress to part 2, you can remind yourself of this whenever you are at the sink.

Position of the Knees

The hip joint doesn't only bend like a hinge, it also lets you rotate your entire leg to the inside or the outside. The rotation of the hip determines whether the knee points forward, to the inside, or to the outside.

Unlike the hip joint, the knee does not rotate inward and outward. It is a hinge, like a book that can open and close. Actually, like a book, the knee can accommodate a little bit of rotation, but repeated or severe rotation will strain the joint. To avoid twisting at the knee when you walk, for example, your knees need to be pointing in the direction that you are walking (that is, straight ahead). More is said about this at the end of the following section about feet.

In addition to being twisted, misaligned knees can be angled inward (knock-kneed) or outward (bowlegged). Both conditions unevenly strain and compress the knee joints and the cartilage inside the knees. These misalignments can begin above the knees, when the thighs are not hanging at the proper angle from the hips because of unbalanced muscle tone in the hip or leg muscles. I know a woman who began ballet as a young child because her family doctor suggested it to help correct her severe condition of knock-knee. Ballet involves frequent use of hip muscles that usually do not function well in a person with knock-knees. This woman is now in her forties and has never had knee pain.

It is also true that knee misalignment can begin below the knees. This happens when the foot does not provide a level base for the lower leg, so the lower leg is tilted too much to the inside or the outside. This tilt can strain the knee joint.

Problems with the Feet

The foot bones form three main arches: an inner longitudinal (lengthwise) arch, an outer longitudinal arch, and a latitudinal (widthwise) arch. Ligaments, with the help of muscles, reinforce the strength of the foot arches. Arches are shock absorbers that cushion the impact of your foot against the ground as you walk. If the arches are either too high or too low, the top of the foot is not level. Because the feet are the foundation on which the legs, and therefore the rest of the body, are balanced, foot problems can cause trouble with alignment throughout the entire body. By the same token, a misalignment of the upper or lower leg can cause you to stand more to the outside or inside of your foot. These conditions create an unbalanced load on the foot arches.

The hips can be aligned so that the entire leg faces forward, or they can be misaligned so that the leg is rotated inward or outward. Since the feet are connected to the legs, they too can point one of three ways. The arches are used best when the feet are pointing straight ahead.

However, when you walk with one or both feet habitually pointing in or out, the arches are compromised and the foot becomes an imbalanced base for the leg. Also, if you walk with your feet pointing in or out, your toes are misaligned. Toes are an important component of your balance. Ideally, they point in the direction in which you are walking.

Stand up and take a look at where your feet are. Most people I see stand with their toes pointing out (sometimes called "duck-footed"). Even if you are not duck-footed, stand with your feet turned out for a minute. Now slowly begin walking forward, keeping your feet turned out. Is your weight distributed evenly over your feet when you walk this way? Notice how most of your weight goes over your big toe, and your little toe is doing no work at all. Look at and feel how this way of walking flattens the arch on the inside of your foot. What will happen to this arch if you spend a lifetime walking this way? Now look at your knees and see how they are not pointing straight ahead. This means that your knees are being twisted and strained with every step. Your feet and knees are not meant to be used this way. The more you can feel and use all of your toes, the better walking will feel.

There is also a connection between collapsed posture of the spine and the condition of the feet. When the waist is collapsed, hip and leg muscle tone is affected all the way down to the feet. Learning to keep your waist as long as possible helps you to center the weight of your body over the middle of each foot. This eases foot strain when you stand. As previously mentioned, psoas muscle tone is essential to having a long waist and lower back. A number of years ago I worked with a woman who had lower back pain, as well as persistent foot pain. She'd had the foot pain for years, despite the use of arch supports in her shoes, exercises, and foot massage. One day I used a hands-on myofascial treatment for her extremely tense psoas muscle to help reduce her lower back pain. When she got up from my treatment table, she shouted, "My feet don't hurt!" I hadn't touched her feet or legs during that treatment. I later taught her exercises for the psoas muscle and gave her two more hands-on treatments. Her foot pain never returned, even after long walks. Repeated events like this convinced me of the importance of the psoas, waist, and lower back to the function of the whole body.

The Head-Neck Relationship

The bones of the neck are called the *cervical spine*. Your head balances at the top of your spine on two rocker-shaped bones at the base of your skull. The rocker shape suggests that the head is intended to move freely, rather than be held in a fixed position. The top vertebra can rotate much more easily than the other vertebrae, and as a result, the head is able to swivel left and right. The top of the neck is approximately at the level of the nose, much higher than many people realize.

Clients often ask me what the "right" position is for the head. There is no right position, because the head needs to be free to move for you to see and hear. The *relationship* of the head to the neck is the issue here, meaning that the head needs to be poised on top of the neck in a way that puts little compression on the neck and the head moves easily in any direction. So regardless of head position at any given moment, it can have a free-floating relationship to the neck.

When the muscle tone of the neck muscles is good, the neck follows the head in movement. To some extent, this sets the muscle tone in the rest of your body, and your joints move freely.

When tension in the neck muscles causes those muscles to grab hold of the head, the head and neck move as if they were welded into a single piece. This restriction of head movement provokes other areas of the body to tighten in response, specifically, the spinal extensors (which go all the way from the neck to the tailbone), the psoas, and the abdominals. When the area between the top of the neck and the back of the skull is compressed, the groundwork is laid for neck pain, headaches, and myriad other muscular tension problems throughout the body.

A man once came to see me because whenever he walked he experienced persistent right foot pain. When I watched him walk, I could see that he twisted his right foot with every step. Further investigation showed that he had a DMP in his lumbar and abdominal muscles that caused misalignment of the entire right leg. At one point, he mentioned that he'd had frequent headaches throughout his life, so I decided to check out his neck. When I had him lie down on his back so I could gently move his head, I found that he could not relax his neck. When he was finally able to let his head move independently from his neck, a remarkable thing happened: he could feel his right waist and hip muscles involuntarily contract and relax. He then remembered that as a baby the muscles on one side of his neck had contracted severely. His mother had stretched his neck daily, and the problem appeared to go away. What really happened is that as a toddler he learned to compensate for an imbalanced head by contracting the muscles of his right lower body. These contractions persisted through his life and eventually caused his right foot pain. He soon developed kinesthetic awareness of his head and neck, and he no longer twisted his right foot with each step. The foot pain was gone.

Problems with the Shoulder Girdle

The shoulder girdle is made up of the two collarbones (*clavicles*), shoulder blades (*scapulae*), arms, and hands. The shoulder girdle is superimposed on the main frame of the skeleton and is therefore not directly involved in maintaining spinal alignment. It is connected to the rest of the skeleton only where the two clavicles join the *sternum* at the top of the chest. The remainder of the shoulder girdle is attached by muscles. Because of its loose attachment, it is able to move freely in many directions.

The arms are connected to the sides of the scapulae. When the alignment of the spine and the shoulder girdle is balanced, the arms hang along the sides of the torso without the need to hold the arms in any particular position. Because the arms are connected to the scapulae at the shoulder joints, the flexibility of the arms depends on the mobility of the scapulae.

Except for direct-impact injuries to the shoulder girdle and some repetitive use injuries, problems with the shoulders, arms, and hands can usually be traced to a musculoskeletal imbalance in the waist and neck areas. Here is how it happens: As mentioned earlier, a DMP in the waist area may cause misalignment of the lumbar spine, hips, or legs, and lower body alignment and muscle use determine the alignment of the upper spine. Since the shoulder girdle depends on the alignment of the upper spine for its own placement, the muscle use of the waist ends up determining the alignment of the shoulders. For example, when the thoracic spinal curve is too concave (caved in) because of a collapsed waist posture, the shoulder girdle slides forward. When this happens, myofascial strain occurs in the arms and hands.

You can test this for yourself by doing a quick experiment. Sit up as tall as possible in a chair, your arms at your sides. Lift both arms in front of you so that your hands are pointing up. Notice how high your arms can reach and how much strain is involved in the movement. Next, slump in your chair so that your upper back is rounded and your chest is caved in. From this slumped position, raise your arms as before. Notice how high your arms will reach and how much strain you feel. Your arms do not rise as easily when your thoracic spine is caved in, because your shoulder joints are restricted. If you maintain a slumped position over time, your shoulders eventually become strained.

The function of the arms and hands is largely dependent on the scapulae and shoulder joints to which they are attached. When shoulder motion is restricted, the arms and hands must strain to make up for the limitations of the shoulders. The result is a variety of chronic strain conditions, such as tendonitis, in the muscles and joints of the upper extremities.

Cumulative Strain in the Limbs: Case Studies

Let's review briefly. When the body center muscles are functioning well, the tone throughout the remainder of the body tends to be balanced automatically. However, if the tone around the body center is either too high or too low, the alignment and mobility of the pelvis and spine are impaired. When this occurs, muscles elsewhere in the body become tense to accommodate for the dysfunction. In addition to this, habitual tension in the neck muscles causes habitual tension in the large muscles of the spine and waist.

As a general rule, when important muscles in your body are not doing their job, other muscles tend to overdo theirs. Your neuromuscular system always uses the most efficient muscular option available for movement. If the body center muscles are either too lax or too inflexible, muscles that represent the second-best option will be recruited. If the second-best option is also not available, the third-best option is used, and so on. Any compensation for tension or slackness in the body center inevitably involves the overuse of muscles farther out toward the extremities. With repetition, this inefficient use of the body becomes habitual, a DMP. Over time, the muscles that compensate for the dysfunction in the body center become strained and hardened. Chronic tension in the arm and leg muscles is therefore the eventual and predictable result of muscle misuse at the body center. The compensations for improper use of the body center follow a fairly predictable order. I have observed the same scenario repeated in hundreds of clients.

I have seen clients who have eliminated pain in one area of their body by correcting the alignment of another. For example, one client's left shoulder pain went away when she learned to walk evenly on her right foot, which involved correcting the alignment of her right leg. Another client eliminated her knee pain when she learned to release her hip and thigh muscles when she stood and walked.

The following two examples describe how muscle tension and misalignment in the middle of the body caused the upper or lower body muscles to tighten. Using limbs that are frequently under muscular and skeletal strain may eventually cause pain symptoms. These problems are often referred to as *overuse problems,* although a more apt expression would be *misuse problems.*

Misuse Problems: Julie

Julie came to see me because she had pain in both hands and wrists, although the right side was worse than the left. Julie worked in an office where she used a computer keyboard at least four hours a day. She reported that her right hand had begun aching about six months before our initial appointment. At first, the ache would go away after about an hour. Within a few months, however, the pain would not go away unless she took an analgesic. After about five months, Julie's left hand and wrist also began to ache. A physician told her that she had tendonitis in both wrists. An ergonomist came to her office to help improve the positioning of the furniture and equipment that she used, but her pain persisted.

When I first saw Julie, she had stopped typing altogether. I could see that her body looked a bit tense. When she moved her right or left arm, I could observe virtually no movement in her scapulae. If she rolled her arms along the floor while lying on an exercise mat, she could feel the pain increasing in her wrists.

I showed Julie a model skeleton and demonstrated where the scapula is and how it moves in conjunction with the arm. I also showed her pictures from an anatomy book to help her to visualize how the scapula is designed to move. I then asked Julie to move her arm and scapula together. She was not able to sense any motion in her scapula as she rolled her arm along the floor; in fact, her scapula was barely moving. Because freedom of movement of the scapula is necessary for easy use of the arm, I began to consider that her lack of shoulder blade motion had something to do with her wrist pain.

The spine moves naturally in relation to the moving scapula, but in Julie's case, the spine was not moving at all. I asked her to perform some basic, gentle movements of her waist, which she found difficult because she was unable to release her lower back muscles. She mentioned that her lower back was often stiff, but it did not really get in her way or cause much pain.

I began to suspect that Julie's hand and wrist pain had little to do with her hands and wrists. As it turned out, she had misalignment and a DMP in her lumbar spine and abdomen that was causing her shoulder muscles to compensate by constantly tightening up. Each scapula was rigidly held in a fixed position so that her shoulders were pulled forward. Because of this shoulder misalignment, her arms did not hang naturally at either side of her body, but instead were pulled around toward the front. The misalignment of the shoulder joint caused arm strain, as she overused her arm muscles to work against the immobility of the scapulae. Since she used her arms so often at the computer keyboard, her arm and wrist muscles became fatigued and painful. When the muscle fatigue became constant, so did the hand and wrist pain.

When I explained the situation to Julie, she had a hard time understanding how her lower back, which hurt very little, had anything to do with her debilitating hand pain. Nevertheless, I showed her corrective exercises for the alignment and muscle use of her body center. Later I showed her movements and techniques for the use of her shoulders.

I saw Julie for a total of eight sessions. By the third session, she noticed that her shoulders moved more freely. By the fourth, the constant stiffness in her back was gone. During the fifth, she was able to sense constant muscle tension in her hands, where she had felt only pain before. By the eighth visit, Julie was able to type at the keyboard without pain. Her recovery resulted from doing exercises for her waist, back, and shoulders, without any specific exercises for her wrists and hands.

Fortunately for Julie, she sought treatment for the pain in her hands and wrists fairly early. I often see clients who have been living with constant arm and hand pain for years, usually taking pain pills and continuing to push themselves to work and move as they have always done. Eventually, when the pain becomes unbearable, they seek help. By this point, the condition has become more difficult to correct, because the passage of time solidifies the dysfunctional movement patterns that initially caused the pain. Nerves and joints have likely become extremely irritated, adding another dimension to the problem. The combination of pain reactions, movement dysfunction, muscle tension, and subsequent mental anxiety further impairs kinesthetic awareness, adding to the severity of the problem. All of a person's reactions and secondary problems must be unraveled before the initial pain can be addressed adequately. A lengthy recovery process can be greatly reduced if a pain problem is addressed soon after it begins.

Misuse Problems: Len

Len came to see me for knee pain that had begun about six months before, at the end of ski season. Len was forty-eight and had done cardiovascular and strength-training exercises for years. The knee pain was now interfering with running and his hopes of skiing the following winter. He noticed that the less he used his legs, the less his knees hurt, but he did not consider becoming inactive an option.

Len's problem turned out to be fairly simple. His waist muscles were so inflexible that he had difficulty bending to the side or rotating at his waist. His hip muscles were constantly contracted, something that felt normal to Len. He was not aware that his leg alignment was distorted until I asked him to stand with his feet parallel to each other. This felt odd to him because he always stood with his feet turned out, duck-footed. With his feet parallel, he said that his knees felt like they were pointing toward each other rather than in the direction of his feet. For the first time, he could actually feel the twisting in his knees as he stood. Remember, knees are made to bend like a hinge, not twist.

When Len walked or ran, the twisting at his knees was amplified, and his knee pain was the result. Inactivity helped simply because his legs were not being moved as much. His problem was not "bad knees," but misalignment of the legs. The repeated motion of running caused a cumulative strain in his knees not because running was bad for them, but because he ran with legs that weren't facing straight ahead.

Len was able to regain his kinesthetic awareness of his lower body by doing exercises I taught him. As this happened, he could feel his hips move more than he ever remembered. As his waist became more flexible, his hip muscles were able to relax and do their job of aligning his legs. Within two months, Len's knee pain was gone. Six months later, I saw him during the ski season, and he was skiing without knee pain.

EXPLORATION 5

Lie on your back with your knees bent and your feet flat on the floor. Place a hand on each side of your pelvis. Drop both of your legs to the left side, keeping your knees bent. Notice how your pelvis rolled to the left when you dropped your legs. Next, slowly return your pelvis and legs to the midline position by initiating the movement with your abdominal muscles. Specifically, you will be using your oblique abdominal muscles, which run diagonally from your chest to the opposite side of your pelvis (see illustration 5.4 on page 88).

These muscles are essential for twisting at the waist. As you return your pelvis and legs to the starting position, think about moving your pelvis and letting your legs follow. Do not use your lower back muscles, and relax your legs as much as possible. If you are unfamiliar with isolating the obliques, you may find yourself using your lower back, hip, and leg muscles instead. If you feel your lumbar curve increasing in height as your pelvis turns, you are using your lower back muscles too much to help you rotate your pelvis.

Alternate to the right and left sides until you can easily feel how your abdominal muscles can cause this turning of your waist.

When you have become familiar with isolating the oblique abdominals, you are ready for a more challenging exploration. This time you will be using the same muscles to roll your upper body a little bit from side to side. Lie on your back with your knees bent and your feet flat on the floor. Cross your arms comfortably over your chest so that your hands are hanging down on each side of your chest.

Slowly roll your upper body back and forth a few inches to the right and left. As much as possible, keep your pelvis from rotating with or against your rib cage. Relax your neck, shoulder, arm, and back muscles so that you are only using your oblique abdominals to turn your chest. This may take a little practice, but it is not impossible. Do not lift your head off the floor; let it roll a little from side to side with your upper body. If your lumbar curve increases as you rotate your chest, you are using your back muscles to rotate instead of your obliques. Relax your lower back as you rotate from side to side.

6

Emotions: The Hidden Cause of Muscular Pain

> Cherish your own emotions and never
> undervalue them.
>
> —*Robert Henri*

SO FAR, I have discussed how you experience pain when parts of your body do not function properly because of injuries, dysfunctional movement patterns, and misalignment. This chapter is intended to give you a basic understanding of the interconnection of the mind, emotions, and body. You will learn about the different ways in which emotional stress can contribute to DMPs, habitually held postures, and muscular pain.

The mind and body are not separate; they are two parts of the whole person. Mental and emotional stress do have physiological effects. If you don't have good kinesthetic awareness, you may have poor emotional receptivity as well. When you become insensitive to your emotions, you miss basic information that you need to make good decisions, and you narrow the range of your personal experiences. This is equivalent to how a lack of kinesthetic awareness can cause you to miss the basic information you need to use your muscles properly.

Psychological stress can combine with neuromuscular and myofascial factors to cause musculoskeletal pain. Pain that has its roots in the function of the psyche is called *psychogenic pain*. I am referring here to actual pain that a person feels in the muscles and joints, not imagined pain.

Moderation and Extremes

To understand how your thoughts and feelings affect your body, it is helpful to think in terms of moderation and extremes. Imagine a continuum, like a number line in mathematics, that extends a great distance in either direction. The entire continuum, from one end to the other, represents how you function. The direction of one extreme represents *underactivity,* while the direction of the other extreme represents *overactivity.* The middle of the continuum represents *moderation.* In general, any function of your mind or body is healthier when it operates in the moderate zone, rather than in either of the extremes.

The body and mind naturally prefer to remain in the moderate area of the continuum. In physiological terms, this preference is known as *homeostasis,* which is a moderate (nonextreme) physiological state that occurs even when a creature is in the presence of an ever-changing external environment. All of the physiological systems in your body are continuously oriented toward homeostasis. For example, your body needs a certain amount of salt to function properly. When there is too much salt, your kidneys get rid of the excess, and when there is too little salt, your kidneys find ways to hold on to it.

From this point of view, illness is the inability of the body to maintain homeostasis in one or more of its systems and adapt to changes. For instance, your body naturally tries to keep your blood pressure within a homeostatic range—neither too high nor too low—but if this range is exceeded because your circulatory system cannot adapt to an ever-changing environment, you may have chronic high blood pressure.

An emotional change occurs simultaneously with biochemical changes in the body. Additionally, a person's ideas and beliefs can lead to feelings and behaviors that affect homeostasis. For example, if a person believes he is inadequate and constantly pressures himself to do more and achieve more, he will become overactive—mentally, physically, and emotionally. Any belief that undermines a person's wholeness will disturb his homeostasis. As you can imagine, personal beliefs and resulting behavior is a huge subject and beyond the scope of this book.

Moderation, or the lack of it, in one's lifestyle directly affects muscle tone. Suppose you are a mentally overactive, time-pressured person who pushes the envelope every day just to keep up with all of the responsibilities of daily life. Sooner or later, your overactivity will lead to tension in your back and shoulder muscles. There is too much work, too much mental effort, and too little restorative time in your life. You are spending too much time on the overactive side of the continuum, and the result is too much tone (tension) in your muscles. If you were to spend some time every day on the underactive side of the continuum, you would automatically bring your muscle tension down to some extent. You could engage in restful activities such as fishing, gardening, napping, or simply stopping to sit and exist. Slowing down your body, relaxing your mind, or both, would help move you toward the middle of the continuum.

On the other hand, if you tend to be underactive due to a sedentary lifestyle, depression, or other reasons, you probably have low muscle tone in your basic postural muscles. This can lead to a collapsed posture with all of the alignment problems that follow. Getting outside more, doing some kind of physical work such as stacking wood or raking the garden, walking, and exercise in general will help increase your overall muscle tone.

In a fundamental way, the psychological or mental state of homeostasis comes about by living with your attention in the present, rather than the past or future. This is because focusing attention too much on what has happened or what might happen creates an extra burden for the mind. Muscle tone and other physiological functions move toward homeostasis when your attention is in the present. Your carriage says something about how present you are *not*. The habitual spinal posture of a future-oriented person will tend to have a more exaggerated lumbar curve, and the habitual posture of a past-oriented person will tend to have a more exaggerated thoracic curve (slouched chest).

Reflexive Emotional Responses

Earlier in this book we discussed how the neuromuscular system controls the skeletal muscles, all of which are potentially within your voluntary control. However, many bodily functions happen unconsciously and are therefore outside of ordinary voluntary control. These functions are carried out by a distinct branch of the nervous system called the *autonomic nervous system*. The autonomic nervous system controls the functioning of your internal organs and glands, such as the digestion of food and the circulation of blood, as well as the emotional functions of aggression and fear.

The autonomic nervous system comprises two smaller branches: the *sympathetic nervous system* and the *parasympathetic nervous system*. The sympathetic system is generally responsible for activating the internal organs, while the parasympathetic system usually calms them. As the requirements of homeostasis or emergency response dictate, the sympathetic and parasympathetic systems can, for example, increase or decrease heart rate, blood pressure, and respiration.

Here is a simplified example of how the sympathetic system can activate the body. If a rabbit encounters a mountain lion, the rabbit's recognition of danger activates its sympathetic nervous system and conditions its actions. The sympathetic nervous system instantaneously sends out the appropriate set of commands to the rabbit's internal organs and muscles, allowing it to either fight, run at top speed, or hold still. When the danger of the lion has passed, the rabbit's sympathetic response subsides and the parasympathetic response returns its physiology to neutral (homeostasis).

In humans, the sympathetic system also responds to the recognition of danger, whether that danger is physical or mental. This means that your sympathetic system will activate if an alligator is chasing you through a swamp or if you are physically safe at home but mentally anxious about the fate of the stock market. Emotional reactions of aggression or fear may also accompany the sympathetic response. After the danger or intense emotional state subsides, the physiological functioning of your body should return to neutral.

Health problems can arise when intense emotional states remain active long after an incident has passed. Ongoing thoughts and feelings, such as hostility or anxiety, constantly trigger the sympathetic system to activate the internal organs and glands. Human beings are adaptable creatures, yet there is a limit to how much the body can endure. Striving to maintain homeostasis in the face of continuous overactivation requires a great deal of energy. When your energy supply gets low enough, you become susceptible to all sorts of illnesses. Simply put, prolonged stress can lead to poor physical health. Ongoing stress can come from two different yet interrelated sources: from living in a stressful environment day after day, or from holding on to upsetting thoughts and emotions long after the initial cause has disappeared.

Neuromuscular Reflexes Triggered by Stress

It may be helpful to think of the sympathetic response and the specific neuromuscular reflexes caused by its reaction to stress in terms of either enlarging or shrinking. In the book *Somatics* (Addison-Wesley, 1988), Thomas Hanna describes how neuromuscular reflexes are activated by emotional stress and how the long-term effects of these reflexes affect posture and flexibility. His explanations are excellent, so I will summarize them briefly here. I recommend *Somatics* to anyone interested in learning more about this subject.

The Extension and Flexion Reflexes

When someone perceives a threat, a neuromuscular reflex occurs that causes her to mobilize for action. This mobilization is accomplished by involuntarily contracting the muscles on the back of the body, which pulls the arms, shoulders, legs, and spine backward in a movement known as *extension*. Hanna referred to this as the green light reflex, and I call it the *extension reflex*. This reflex has its roots in the natural muscular reaction found in all healthy babies, known as the Landau reaction. The Landau reaction can be seen when you hold a baby in the air with your hands under her belly; her back arches, her head lifts up, and her knees straighten. The extension reflex is the "fight" part of the so-called fight-or-flight response. It can be triggered by any sudden urge to fight back, as well as by time pressure, overwork, and stress in general.

In contrast, if someone experiences fear in response to a perceived threat, an involuntary protective response can occur. This is a full body muscular reflex that generally pulls the body in toward a fetal position, a movement known as *flexion*. Hanna referred to this as the red light reflex, and I call it the *flexion reflex*. This reflex is based in the withdrawal response found in all animals. The withdrawal response induces many physiological changes, including the guarding of the vital organs by involuntarily contracting the muscles on the front of the body. The flexion reflex is the "flight" part of the fight-or-flight response. It can be triggered by hearing an unexpected loud noise, as well as by feeling anxious, overwhelmed, or pressured.

The extension and flexion reflexes represent two distinct neuromuscular reactions that we use automatically and habitually to adapt to stress in our environment. Some people are prone toward extension, others toward flexion. There are also many people who hold themselves in a posture that combines these two reflexes.

When teaching group classes, I often use a simple activity to illustrate the difference between flexion and extension. I ask half of the class to exaggerate the flexion reflex by intentionally tightening all of the muscles along the front of their bodies. I ask the other half of the class to exaggerate the extension reflex by tightening all of the muscles along the back of their bodies. After they hold themselves in these positions for a minute, I ask them to stand up while still holding their exaggerated positions, walk around the room, and pay attention to how their bodies feel. After a few minutes, I ask them to walk up to others in the group at random and introduce themselves, while observing how they feel emotionally when interacting with others from their postures. The comments people make about this exercise are often remarkable. Those who exaggerate the flexion reflex often say they feel weak, embarrassed, afraid, intimidated, and lowly. People who exaggerate the extension reflex tend to feel proud, pushy, strong, aloof, and confident. They can usually feel the emotional effect of these exaggerated postures, even after only a few minutes. Intentionally exaggerating a posture or muscle tension amplifies the kinesthetic sense, making both the physical and emotional feelings associated with the body position more obvious.

Although significant, these responses are really not too surprising. All of us naturally know how a person's carriage suggests certain character traits. This is why people around the world enjoy watching clowns. A skilled clown can exaggerate body postures and facial expression to instantly convey the feelings of his or her character without saying a word to the audience. We know what the character is feeling because his body language tells us.

I sometimes have participants resume their exaggerated postures, but this time using only about 5 percent of their muscular force. This lets them experience a more hidden and subtle reflexive posture that more closely approximates how it would feel to have habitual muscle tension for years and years. As we saw in chapter 2, a person with poor carriage and muscle tension eventually becomes unable to sense these things clearly, because his kinesthetic awareness is distorted from receiving the same input over and over. Typically, such a person also loses the recognition of the emotional feelings related to his habitual posture: emotional insensitivity parallels kinesthetic insensitivity. If your body is stuck in a rigid posture, your emotional experience will diminish because you will have difficulty feeling the emotions in your body.

Neuromuscular Reflexes in Daily Life: Joan

In previous chapters, we explored the protective response of neuromuscular reflexes when triggered by physical pain. The neuromuscular reflexes of flexion and extension, however, can also be triggered without physical impact, injury, or pain. They can be activated wholly as a result of the mind and emotions. In daily life, most people do not encounter overt physical danger. The flexion and extension reflexes can be activated by the simple stresses of daily life and profoundly affect both body alignment and psychological self-image. Reflexive reactions can occur from head to toe. You might feel the tension in your neck, your lower back, your feet, or anywhere else in your body.

Imagine that you have been working for the same company for twenty years. During that time, the company has been successful, and you have established a secure and comfortable position for yourself within the organization. One day, you come to work and discover that your company is being acquired by a larger corporation. The new management is looking for ways to cut costs and has decided to downsize your company to save money. You know that you could lose your job and some of your fellow workers could lose theirs.

This situation is stressful and threatening because you are concerned for the financial and physical well-being of yourself and your entire family. This anxiety activates your sympathetic nervous system. A near-accident on the freeway, where you swerve out of the way just in time, is also a threat to the well-being of yourself and your family; your sympathetic nervous system would be activated in the same way. In the freeway example, though, you react reflexively, without thinking, to protect yourself. The threat is clear, and it is resolved quickly, one way or the other. In the case of your employment status, however, the threat is ongoing and unresolved. You are in doubt about what is going to happen to you, and you have no definitive way of finding out. This stressful situation may continue for weeks or even months before you find out whether you will keep your job. The absence of resolution creates a chronic feeling of anxiety. You do not have a chance to relax and recover from the emotional threat because your sympathetic system does not have a chance to calm down.

A case study from my professional experience can help to illustrate this point. Some years ago, I worked with Joan, a middle-aged woman who had chronic neck stiffness and pain. She had tried spinal adjustments, massage treatments, and a special pillow, yet she continued to have neck pain. She told me that the stiffness had been intermittent when she was in her twenties, and she had just ignored it. Now that she was in her forties, the pain was constant.

I could see in Joan's posture that her head was pulled forward and down and that her chest had a subtle caved-in appearance. While she was lying flat on the treatment table, I moved her head gently. I felt a tremendous resistance in her neck muscles when I attempted to move her head either backward or up. Furthermore, Joan could not rotate her head very far to either side without pain.

When I asked Joan to do some simple waist movements, she was unable to use her abdominal muscles properly. As we continued to explore further, she was able to feel that her abdominal muscles were in a constant state of contraction, even when she was lying still. Interestingly, she had never noticed this tension before.

I showed her a few exercises for learning how to relax her abdominals, which she was able to do well. At the end of the first session, she was able to turn her head twice as far to both sides. When I gently pulled on her head, she felt her entire neck lengthen, something that would have been impossible before this session. All of these changes occurred as a result of using and releasing her abdominal muscles.

Joan's neck pain and stiffness were caused by a prolonged activation of the flexion reflex, which includes the abdominal muscles. When the abdominal muscles contract reflexively, the rib cage is pulled down toward the pelvis. The head is pulled forward and held down by the fallen rib cage. Since Joan's neck muscles were contracting as part of the flexion reflex, this reflex needed to be turned off to let her neck relax. Relaxing the abdominal muscles was the key.

I explained to Joan how fear can activate the flexion reflex and how this affects the alignment by caving in the chest. Joan said that her mother's posture was even more extreme than hers and that her mother tended to be full of fears and anxieties. Joan asked if this situation could be genetic. I told her that blaming genetics avoids the real issue, which is that she had beliefs about herself and the world that created habitual fear and anxiety. Throughout her life, Joan had subconsciously learned psychological attitudes that directly affected her muscles and carriage.

Joan confirmed this fact during one of her subsequent appointments. She had been practicing exercises at home that increased her kinesthesia of all the major muscles in the front of her body. I had asked her to try to notice if and when these muscles would contract during the course of her day. The first time she noticed these muscles tightening was while she was entering traffic on the freeway. Joan worked as a schoolteacher, and she was now aware of her muscles contracting while at school. She noticed that her neck and abdominal muscles would tighten up when she was confronting one of her students. Over the next few days, she realized that these muscles were contracting almost all day long, even when nothing particularly stressful appeared to be happening.

Joan understood that she had a subconscious habit of tightening her abdominals whether or not she was in an obviously stressful situation. When she *was* in a stressful situation, the muscle contractions were even stronger. Now she was aware of the hidden stress that was almost continuously present in her body. She realized that the reflex causing her chronic muscle tension was being triggered by her own habitual fears and anxieties.

As Joan's case shows, thoughts and beliefs can fall into habitual patterns, just like muscles. Underlying mental attitudes—for example, about competence, our importance to others, and the hospitality of the world—are programmed into us. These beliefs influence our perception of our whole self. Just as dangers in the external environment can activate an emergency response from your nervous system, perceived threats within your mind can do the same. In fact, completely imaginary fears can activate the sympathetic system as effectively as real danger. A rhinoceros charging at you can be a source of serious stress. The belief that you will always fail, no matter how hard you try, can be just as serious. Both can activate neuromuscular reflexes that cause the muscles along the entire length of your body to tighten.

When emotional stress results in chronic muscle tension, the reflexive reaction of the muscles becomes habitual. The kinesthetic dysfunction that typically follows any kind of long-term, involuntary muscular contraction will likely come into play. Even if the emotional circumstances that initially activated the muscle reflexes have been resolved, the DMPs can persist. In other words, you may still have some muscle habits to contend with.

In my practice, I have seen many people like Joan, in whom some combination of the flexion and extension reflexes have caused constant muscular pain. Occasionally, these people can learn to turn off the muscle contractions intentionally after only one or two visits, thereby dramatically reducing their pain. All they need is someone to make them aware of the constant muscle contractions, because they can no longer sense them on their own. They can improve their kinesthesia easily by practicing movement explorations and exercises that release their muscles. In other cases, however, these reflexes cannot be addressed quite so easily. The difference is that some people continue to activate their muscular reflexes by the distressing thoughts and feelings they have every day.

Psychogenic Pain

Years ago, I began to notice something surprising that would occasionally happen to clients with very tense muscles and specific pain. After a number of treatment sessions, these clients would return with completely relaxed muscles, yet they were still suffering from the same pain. For some reason, relaxing their tense muscles had absolutely no effect on their pain. They also had no evidence of any structural problems.

One such person was Donna, who had tension and recurring pain in her shoulders. At first, she was incapable of relaxing her shoulders. After a number of treatments involving hands-on therapy and corrective movement exercise, which she also practiced at home, I noticed that the tension was completely gone from both of her shoulders. Yet she continued to experience pain in exactly the same muscles.

Early in my career, when I worked as a massage therapist, I gave thousands of treatments to people with tense shoulder muscles. Often, if I began working with a person who had hard and inflexible shoulders, they would be at least a little softer and more pliable by the end of an hour. Usually, the person would get up from the massage table and say that his or her shoulders felt less painful and tense. There was an obvious relationship between the muscles relaxing and the pain decreasing. How could I explain Donna's situation, in which muscle relaxation had no effect on her muscular pain? Her muscle pain was being generated by some process of her psyche and mind, so simply relaxing the muscles did not get to the root of the problem.

Another peculiar phenomenon I experienced was when, after a treatment that released contracted muscles, a client would return for the next treatment and tell me that the original pain had gone, but now an entirely new pain had developed in a different location. One explanation is that when the muscles in one area are released, it can alter alignment and cause muscles somewhere else to pull in a new way. However, there are instances where this explanation makes no sense at all.

A perfect example of this was Lily, who came to see me for help with neck pain. At the close of the session, she said that her neck was almost free of pain. She called me the next day, though, and told me that she had woken up with such intense pain in her left foot that she could barely walk. The foot pain was entirely new, and she had felt nothing unusual or painful in the foot the day before.

Lily's case represents a bodily pain problem that originates in the mind. Her pain was real physical pain, not imaginary pain. But instead of the pain being caused by strain from poor alignment, muscle tension, or neuromuscular or myofascial reaction to an injury, it had a psychological origin. Lily had suppressed her emotional feelings to the extent that she actually lost awareness of them. Her neck pain was the result of suppressing her emotional awareness. My treatment relaxed her neck but did not give her any awareness of the emotional cause of the pain. So her nervous system moved the pain down to her foot. This notion has been understood by traditional Asian doctors for thousands of years. They know that emotions are not separate from the body, and therefore suppressing one's awareness of emotions is harmful to the body. It is really that simple.

A modern-day champion of the idea that the psyche can be the cause of musculoskeletal pain is John Sarno, MD. In his books *Healing Back Pain* (Warner Books, 1991) and *The Mindbody Prescription* (Warner Books, 1998), Sarno goes into detail about the diagnostic and treatment methods he has used, with notable success, for musculoskeletal pain. He refers to this kind of pain as psychogenic, which literally means "psychologically caused."

In his books, Sarno gives a plausible explanation for psychogenic pain. He suggests that localized oxygen deprivation can cause a physiological change that irritates pain receptors in a specific area. The oxygen deprivation is caused by the constriction of arteries around muscles, joints, and nerves in response to suppressed emotion. In my opinion, this response originates in the sympathetic nervous system, which controls both the arteries and the emotions. In any event, as long as a person's attention is preoccupied with physical pain, she will tend to be distracted from her underlying emotional unrest, which she has suppressed. Therefore, the solution to this type of pain is to mentally recognize that the physical pain is a distraction and then to regain awareness of one's feelings. Sarno describes a practical method for accomplishing this in his books.

Holding On to Feelings

Emotional feelings occur in waves, just as movement in the ocean occurs in waves. An ocean wave is a movement that passes through the water; an emotion is a movement that passes through a person. The surface of the ocean can be calm until a wave passes through and disrupts that calm. After the wave has passed, the surface will be calm again. Similarly, emotions can emerge, rise, fall, and then fade away. You can see the transient nature of emotions most easily in young children. They can experience an emotion such as anger or sadness and then five minutes later play happily again. They experience their emotions as they occur, and when the emotions are finished, they let go of them. In this respect, adults can learn something from children.

Many adults have been conditioned by their lives to ignore or interfere with the natural ebb and flow of emotions. This interference develops as a way to adapt to difficult or dysfunctional emotional environments they experience, particularly in childhood.

Typically, adults interfere with the natural flow of emotions in one of two ways. One is to continue to think about and relive an emotion, which prevents that emotion from fading away naturally. The other is to suppress or deny an emotion so that it is ignored. Both of these reactions are sources of psychogenic pain.

When you hold on to your feelings, the emotional wave rises but does not fall and move on. The wave is suspended at some point in its progress, so the energy of the emotion does not fade. This happens when the mind continues to dwell on an emotional experience, going over it again and again. This continual thinking generates the emotion long after the original event that caused it has passed.

As you may have guessed by now, the mind and the psyche are not separate. Simply put, the mind thinks and the psyche feels. Your thoughts affect your feelings, and your feelings affect your thoughts.

When an emotion arises, the sympathetic nervous system is engaged. When an emotional wave does not naturally complete itself, the sympathetic system remains active and continues to trigger muscular reflexes. If a person keeps thinking about a past incident, he will keep experiencing any unresolved emotions related to that incident. If this happens, there is a potential for a constant involuntary muscle contraction.

Whenever pain is sufficiently intense, it activates the pain reflex, as in response to physical injury (see chapter 4). This reflex causes muscles to contract involuntarily. Additionally, the muscular pain that results from habitual flexion or extension reflexes can also trigger the pain reflex. This is what happened to a client of mine named Jim, who proclaimed that his son-in-law was the cause of his stiff neck. Jim's daughter, son-in-law, and two grandchildren had come to live with him and his wife. His daughter was in college, and his son-in-law was out of work. Jim was retired and liked to spend time at home, working on the house and the garden. He told me how aggravated he was with his daughter's husband, who lounged around the house all day, apparently unconcerned about finding a job. He considered his son-in-law to be a lazy freeloader and resented him because of it.

This situation went on for months. Jim became furious whenever he talked about it. I asked him why he did not ask his daughter and her family to move out. He replied that he and his wife felt responsible for their grandchildren, and they could not imagine what it would be like for them if the whole family were thrown out. In particular, Jim's wife wanted to help her daughter's family by providing free room and board until the daughter's college graduation, which was still a year away.

Jim's neck and shoulders were continually tense and sore. He was not denying his feelings—he knew he was angry. But since he would not accept the situation as it was, the anger was reactivated nearly every day. He would not accept the fact that his daughter had married such a lazy person, and he would not accept the fact that his house would continue to be a home to his daughter's family for at least another year. Nor would he accept the fact that his son-in-law could get away with not working for a living or the double bind in which Jim found himself.

I did not have any easy answers to Jim's domestic crisis. But it was clear to both of us that his neck and shoulders were constantly tensing as a result of the anger he felt. Being angry once did not make his muscles chronically tense; being angry all the time did. Jim was holding on to his anger, mentally replaying all the irritating scenes, and justifying to himself why he was angry. His sympathetic nervous system was constantly activated, resulting in the reflexive muscle tightening in his neck and back. As long as his emotional tension continued, his muscular tension continued. Jim's anger was like a wave that never completed itself. He could not resolve his wave of anger, so his emotions continued to activate his sympathetic system and the neuromuscular reflexes, which continued to cause pain.

I explained that if he could accept his emotional situation and move on, the emotional wave would be able to dissipate and the sympathetic reflexes would turn off. This is what happened after Jim understood that he was not a victim of circumstance but had a choice to either accept the situation or not. When he acknowledged that his priority was to help his grandchildren and that he was choosing to help them, he was able to intentionally stop fighting the circumstances that went along with that choice. It dawned on him that he was torturing himself by hanging on to the emotions that caused the pain in his neck and shoulders. After Jim let go of this constant irritation and anger, the neck and shoulder pain disappeared.

Denial of Feelings

The second source of emotional interference and psychogenic pain is not as obvious as holding on to your emotions. It is hiding from feelings by denying or suppressing them.

To deny a feeling, your mind intervenes with certain thoughts that take your attention away from it. For example, your feelings might be hurt as the result of an argument with someone. You might tell yourself, "I shouldn't be hurt. I don't like feeling this way." If you can use these thoughts to move your attention away from your hurt feelings, then you will stop feeling hurt.

In the short run, suppressing certain feelings can be an effective strategy for dealing with situations that are emotionally overwhelming. For example, bypassing your emotional reactions can be useful in an emergency so you can do what is needed, such as run from a burning building. As a way of life, however, habitually denying emotions is harmful. If you began denying emotions as a child, you will have become an expert by the time you are an adult. You will deftly be able to deny certain feelings the instant they arise, before you are even aware they exist. If someone then tries to talk to you about these denied emotions, you will not know what he is talking about. How can you, when you don't know they exist?

What is so bad about blocking out certain feelings? What about the old saying, "What you don't know won't hurt you"? In terms of denying your feelings, what you don't know may hurt you because suppressing your feelings can have a negative effect on your health. The ability to respond emotionally is an integral part of who you are. When an emotion arises, it exists. Once it exists, it cannot be snuffed out. Just like a wave on the ocean, the emotion has its own force and momentum that is directed toward completing itself. If you have developed the ability to suppress your emotions at the beginning of the wave, you may believe that the emotion simply goes away. In reality, it is *you* who goes away. The energy of the emotion still exists and still produces physiological effects.

An emotion denied continues to have a force in your psyche, and that force is aimed at resolving the emotion. Lack of emotional resolution acts like an irritant on the psyche, even if you are unaware of the emotion. Moreover, the psychological irritation is also a physiological irritation (remember, the psyche and the body are not separate). This is how a person can develop muscular pain symptoms as the result of denied or suppressed emotions. The connection between suppressed emotions and physical pain is not a new idea. For thousands of years, traditional cultures around the world have seen emotions as the source of some physical pain.

Emotions occur in response to the internal environment of your mind and body and the external environment of the outside world. They are information about how you feel about events and what you want to do about them. This information helps you to navigate successfully through life. If you cut off your connection to your emotions, you lose a large chunk of the information base for living your life. In addition to having emotions, you have the capacity to be logical and reasonable, which is also needed to get through life successfully. Emotions are appropriate and necessary in most situations; logic and reason are needed occasionally. If you habitually use your rational mind to deal with situations that need an emotional response, or if you habitually use your mind to deny your emotions, you will lose touch with your emotional intelligence and set yourself up for psychogenic pain.

Denial of emotion is common. Have you ever told someone (or been told by someone), "You shouldn't be angry; it won't do any good"? This is the mind rationalizing the suppression of anger. But it doesn't matter whether your mind thinks you *should* be angry or not. If you're angry, you're angry, regardless of what your mind thinks about it. When an emotion begins, a bodily process is activated. Your mind is capable of suppressing the effects of those processes to some extent by diverting your attention, but the memory of the emotion never dissipates completely. That memory remains dormant in the body and operates as an invisible cause of pain.

When you suppress a strong emotion, there is a potential for a physical reaction in almost every physiological system in your body. In particular, suppressed emotion can cause pain in muscles and joints. After that pain begins, you may tighten your muscles reflexively in reaction to it (the pain reflex). Now there are two causes of pain: the original psychogenic pain and the tension of the pain reflex. For example, I have worked with people who had back pain and experienced definite relief from using exercises or hands-on treatments, but they continued to have some underlying pain that would not go away. In these cases, the muscle relaxation took away the pain caused by the pain reflex, but they still needed to address their underlying emotional stress to feel complete relief.

Mental Anticipation of Pain

A third area in which emotions can cause physical pain is the mental anticipation of pain. This occurs when someone has experienced pain from an injury or neuromuscular reaction in the past and continues to *expect* the pain to be there. Expecting pain to occur has the potential to make it occur. I am referring here to a natural expectation of pain based on past experience.

If you experience pain every time you raise your left arm above your shoulder, you naturally expect to feel the same pain when you raise your arm again. Underneath this expectation is your memory of pain. This memory causes your muscles to contract, which then can cause the same pain every time you raise your arm over your shoulder. So your anticipation of pain makes it more likely that you will end up having pain. Frequently, people mistake this situation for one in which there is an actual structural problem or injury.

Richard provides a good example of this. Richard was forty-five years old when he first came to see me. He had pain in his entire back, his neck and shoulders, his hips, and his knees. He had tried many kinds of exercises, treatments, and drugs, but he continued to experience increasing pain. He drove long distances for his job. He found that he could only sit in his car for an hour before he had to stop to stretch and walk around.

I taught Richard a variety of exercises, and over the subsequent months, his back pain gradually disappeared. He came for appointments infrequently for the next few years, during which time the pain in his shoulders, neck, and hips completely disappeared. He told me that he was feeling great and was finally able to go on long car rides without any lower back pain.

There was only one area left that still hurt Richard, and that was in his knees. One indication of his knee stiffness was that he was unable to kneel on the floor and sit back with his buttocks getting anywhere close to touching his heels. Now that his back was feeling good again, Richard wanted to do more vigorous exercise. I suggested walking, but he could not walk more than a quarter of a mile before his knees started "killing" him. Jogging was totally out of the question, and he never squatted.

I assessed Richard again and could find no evidence of a myofascial cause for his knee pain. His doctors had given him inconclusive information. One doctor had diagnosed chondromalacia, which is a softening of the knee cartilage. Richard was worried that he had worn out his knees.

I told him that I could find nothing unusual about his knees. His alignment was excellent. He had balanced muscle tone in his legs, and there was no indication of problems with connective tissue adhesions. In my opinion, it was unlikely that he had real knee damage.

I noticed that Richard was extremely tentative whenever he had to do a movement that involved bending his knees. For example, when I asked him to show me how far he could go toward sitting back on his heels, he was unable to relax while doing so, even when it did not hurt. He said that he could not relax because he knew he would feel a sharp pain at some point.

Richard said he had gone through all of the therapy and drugs that his doctors had suggested for his knees, but nothing had changed. The irritation level in his knees fluctuated from day to day. He could not definitely link the level of irritation to his level of activity. For example, on some days, when he barely walked at all, his knees were still very irritated, yet on other days when he walked more, they were less so. Because his knee pain was so inconsistent, I began to doubt there was any injury in either of his knees.

I asked Richard to try an experiment, to assume for one month that there was nothing wrong with his knees and that the pain was due to anticipation of pain or some other emotional pressure. Keep in mind that I had good reason to conclude that his knees were sound and would not be injured. This suggestion was a bit difficult for him to accept, because he was still afraid he would really damage his knees. I told him there was either something wrong with his knees or there wasn't. If his knees were damaged, he had been damaging them all along by the type of work he does, and one more month and a little more walking would not make much difference. If his knees were actually okay, he had nothing to worry about.

Richard accepted my reasoning and decided to give it a try. His assignment was to take a walk every day, and when he felt knee pain, he was to remind himself that there was nothing wrong with his knees. We went over the list of logical reasons that indicated that his knees were healthy. He was free to repeat the list to himself as much as he wanted. The list would help him deal with the fear that he might really be doing damage to his knees by walking and also to short-circuit his expectation of pain.

Richard called me two weeks later and told me that he had been walking every day and his legs did not hurt any worse as a result. He went so far as to suggest that they even felt a little better. Because of this, he had begun to refute the idea that his knees were damaged. Until his recent experiment with walking, Richard had reached the point where he would decide on where to go to dinner with his wife based on how far he would need to walk from the car to the restaurant. But now he could walk three miles and did not feel any greater knee pain as a result; in fact, the pain was slightly less.

For years, Richard's expectation of knee pain had caused muscle contractions that ultimately led to that pain, like a self-fulfilling prophecy. Encouraged by his initial success with this mental approach to his pain, he continued to remind himself that his knees were okay as he took his daily walks. He called me about six months later to say that he had gradually regained the ability to bend his knee farther. He had just reached the point where he could kneel on the floor and sit back on his heels without pain. He walked as much as he wanted and had no more irritation in his knees.

Allowing Your Feelings

Some people with whom I discuss the subject of psychogenic pain are skeptical. Some think I'm talking about some sort of unfounded pop psychology. Others think that I must be talking only about people with a clinical mental illness. Of course, neither is the case. The fact is that the emotions are part of both the mind and the body. The effect that feelings have on your body is only difficult to see when you deny your awareness of either your emotions or your body. It is hard to understand something that is hidden from your awareness, yet accepting the idea of psychogenic pain is not a matter of belief. It is a matter of sensible evaluation: how your pain problem presents itself, diagnostic test results, outcomes from previous therapies, all combined with an understanding of how the mind and body are inseparable.

Accepting What Is: Greg

People often ask me if they need to get rid of all of their stress to make their pain go away. Getting rid of stress is a virtual impossibility and not even advisable. In fact, general wisdom now says that a moderate amount of stress is necessary to stay healthy. Admittedly, some stressful situations are more difficult to deal with than others, but as a general rule, it is your *reaction* to stress that is the problem, not the stress itself. Stressful situations evoke an emotional response. If you deny or ignore your emotional responses, you may avoid feeling the turmoil, but this suppression of emotion can eventually cause physical pain.

However, if you react to stress by allowing yourself to feel your emotions as they come and go, they will eventually dissipate. Essentially, you are allowing your feelings to be what they are, without rationalizing, denying, or changing them. This is simply a matter of accepting the reality of the situation, accepting *what is.* You may experience some temporary emotional pain, but your emotional energy is not blocked and therefore does not cause unnecessary physical pain.

This is what Greg learned when I treated him for lower back pain. Greg was forty-four and had had back pain for years. In the past, he'd undergone chiropractic manipulation and massage therapy, neither of which had a lasting effect. He also learned stretching exercises and yoga, both of which made him feel better in general but did not alleviate his back pain. When I first saw him, he told me that he felt like he was getting old. Not surprisingly, he was discouraged that all his efforts to find pain relief had failed.

I noticed that Greg's body was in a collapsed posture. Since correcting muscle use and misalignment often quickly solves lower back pain, I taught him exercises (many of which are in this book) that gave him a sense of how to support his spine properly. After a few weeks, his carriage was becoming much more upright. He felt great about this and was able to breathe more deeply and easily than before. However, he still had the same pain in his lower back.

When I mentioned to Greg that emotional pressure from denied feelings had the potential to cause back pain, he perked up right away. It made perfect sense to him. Greg's advantage was that he already had a sense that he was not dealing well with his emotions. I had two suggestions for him. First, he needed to challenge his own idea that something was "wrong" with his back by remembering that his alignment had improved and he had no evidence of a structural back problem. Second, I asked him to be on the lookout for any natural emotions that he avoided feeling.

Greg called me two weeks later and said that his back pain was gone. Relieving his back pain was fantastic, but he was even more excited about the emotional relief he was feeling. He saw that ignoring and suppressing his anger had become a habit. When he just let himself feel when he was angry, the emotion was no longer a problem. He realized that being angry does not require acting out. He could just let himself feel what he was feeling, and that feeling would eventually fade away. Greg's story lends truth to the old saying, "What you resist will persist." By attempting to avoid his real feelings of anger, they became stronger. Paradoxically, when Greg simply let himself feel angry, he became a less angry person.

He said that he had been trying to relax for as long as he could remember and had been telling himself that he should not get so angry about things. When he was aware of being angry, he would try to relax, thereby further avoiding his feelings. By telling himself that he *should* relax and *should not* be the way he was, Greg had a basic conflict, because he was habitually, chronically, not accepting *what is*. For years, he had not experienced his anger in the present tense because he had been too busy trying to make it go away or ignoring it. The result of this frequent denial of reality was chronic back pain.

Your Emotional Intelligence

Your body, psyche, and mind work together as a team, with information constantly passing back and forth between them. Together they attempt to maintain health and well-being. I had a personal experience a number of years ago that clued me in to how immediately and securely the body, psyche, and mind are connected to each other.

At the time, I had been studying a strenuous dance technique. One day I was at home practicing a movement that involved squatting low while spinning around very fast, then standing up quickly. In the middle of my practice session, I received a phone call. I was expecting an important call, so I stopped for a few minutes to speak on the phone. The call lasted about five minutes; then I returned to my practice.

As soon as I squatted down, I got a shooting pain in my left knee. The pain was so severe that it almost knocked me over. When I squatted down and stood up slowly, I could feel a sharp pain at a certain point of knee flexion (bending). The pain felt as if it were coming from somewhere inside the knee joint. I thought that perhaps my muscles had cooled down during the phone call, even though in all my years of athletics and dance, I had never had a pain come on so suddenly from taking a break. I did about five minutes of gentle exercises to lengthen my leg muscles and warm up my legs. I slowly squatted again, and the pain was unchanged. I deeply massaged the tendons and muscles all around the knee joint for another few minutes. Once more, I squatted down, and the knee pain was still there, as intense as ever.

I began to worry. Maybe I had injured my knee doing all this spinning around, jumping, and squatting. But I had not felt anything out of the ordinary before the pain started. One thing was sure: I could not continue to practice with such pain in my knee.

I sat down and tried to figure out what had happened. For some reason, I began thinking about the phone call. The call had brought up an issue about which I was feeling very insecure, a situation over which I had no control. As I sat there, I realized that I had been really disturbed by the call. As I remembered the conversation, I also remembered clearly the point at which I'd had a strong pang of fear. After that, I felt nothing in particular. In fact, by the time I hung up the phone I had forgotten the issue altogether.

At least, I *thought* I had forgotten it. I had interrupted the emotional wave as soon as the feelings of fear and insecurity emerged. My mind had done such a good job of blocking out my feelings that while I was talking, I had no sense of fear at all. I was amazed that I could have so effectively hidden such a strong feeling from myself.

I began to make a connection. Since my knee began to hurt after the phone call and it turned out that I was upset about the call, maybe the knee pain came from the suppressed feelings of insecurity. I closed my eyes and focused my attention on my feelings of fear and uncertainty. I simply let myself feel the feelings I had just uncovered. I talked to myself, saying, "I am afraid of what is going to happen because I don't have control of the situation. I am afraid, yet I am going forward."

This could seem a little absurd, to sit and repeat out loud that I was feeling afraid and vulnerable. However, it is even more absurd that I denied the reality of my feelings in the first place. Repeating the emotional facts to myself was an antidote for the habit of hiding from my real feelings. Talking to myself was a simple way to bring me up-to-date on what was really happening.

This impromptu self-therapy session lasted no more than five minutes. After that, I stood up and decided to try squatting one more time. I squatted down and had absolutely no pain in my left knee. I spun around a few times in the squatting position and still felt nothing. I then resumed my practice session, which continued at full speed for another hour. I felt no more pain in my knee. In fact, I never felt it again.

That experience gave me new appreciation for how closely the psyche and the body are linked. Our emotions are a force, and in a sense, demand respect. If we ignore them entirely, they come out in some other way. Emotions are part of our vital energy, and to cut off that energy is not only a disservice to ourselves, but unhealthy as well.

Cutting yourself off from emotional feelings cuts off your access to emotional energy, leaving only your rational mind to provide the information to deal with a given situation. Instead of experiencing certain feelings as problems, you can experience them as energy you can use to give yourself the strength you need to move forward. For example, if you are feeling anxious about a presentation you are about to give, experience the actual feeling of energy in your body at that moment instead of dwelling on your fears. If the energy gets blocked, it will feel like anxiety; if it is not blocked, it will feel like enthusiasm. Emotional energy is harnessed by being in the present, allowing feelings to run their course without suppressing them or reacting to them. This may not seem so easy, but it is ultimately easier than living with pain.

People can go through life with "emotional suppression" as their default setting. The rational mind can take over, and life goes on. In fact, some people can become very successful in business or other pursuits if they are not distracted by their emotions. Emotions can seem out of one's control and can interfere with a busy schedule. Rational thought, on the other hand, is predictable and can actually help a person manage a hectic and busy life. The only problem with this way of living is that it is fundamentally unhealthy; your feelings are a large part of your whole self.

We live in a society that believes the rational is more important than the emotional. In general, one could say that mental strengths tend to be valued more than emotional strengths. Intelligence quotient (IQ) is valued more than emotional quotient (EQ). This is not to say that we disregard emotions altogether, but they take a back seat to reason. This is not balanced, just as it is not balanced to always place more weight on one leg than the other.

Sorting Out the Causes of Pain: Karen

We are now accumulating a large collection of possible reasons, other than structural damage, for someone to have musculoskeletal pain. The cause could be a reflexive muscular reaction from an injury, DMPs, poor alignment and body use, kinesthetic dysfunction, or how emotions are handled. It could also be any combination of these. The way to find the cause or causes of your own muscular pain is to understand as much as possible about how all the possible causes can occur.

In general, the more factors that are behind your pain, the longer it will take to correct the situation. Each cause must be undone in order to progress further. When someone has most or all of the previously mentioned causes occurring together, it is easy for her to be confused about where to begin.

Karen's case is a good example of muscular pain combined with psychogenic pain. She was a violinist who felt a sharp pain in her left thumb when she played for any length of time. I found that she had been contracting two different muscles in the back of her left shoulder to such an extent that they were painful to touch. She had kinesthetic dysfunction in these muscles that was fairly typical. My hands-on treatment helped her both to sense the habitual muscle tension and to relax the muscles. I taught her exercises to practice at home so she could control the muscle tension in her shoulder.

Karen called me a week later to say that the pain was gone from her thumb. She was now aware of her body use and the relaxation in her shoulder when she was playing her violin. It sounded as though she had solved the problem easily.

She returned two months later because she was feeling left thumb pain again. She said that she had been practicing quite extensively for upcoming performances. She was still practicing the exercises I'd taught her and paying attention to relaxing her shoulder when she played. I checked the shoulder muscles that had been the problem the last time, and they did not feel nearly as tense as they had before. She was able to relax them fairly easily. As I was puzzling over why her hand pain had returned despite doing the exercises and her ability to better relax her shoulder, she told me something very interesting. She woke up one morning with hand pain even though she had not played the violin for two days previously. Instead, she had been studying for her college midterm exams and had spent those two days studying. She thought it was strange that her hand hurt despite her rest from practicing.

I asked Karen if she had been uptight while studying. She replied that she was taking two extra courses that semester and was just barely able to keep up with her workload. Yes, she was very anxious the whole time she was studying. She added that she was a perfectionist and typically put a lot of pressure on herself to do the best job possible.

Until this point, I had linked Karen's left hand pain to habitual shoulder tension while playing the violin. With this new information, however, it was clear that her pain was not only due to musculoskeletal causes. Her handling of emotional stress was also affecting her hand. Karen contacted me one week later and told me that the thumb pain had gone away hours after her last visit and had not returned.

A Chicken or Egg Situation

In many situations, it can be difficult to know which came first, the chicken or the egg. Does emotional dysfunction cause the pain and contracted muscles, or do contracted muscles, poor kinesthesia, and pain cause emotional dysfunction? The answer to both questions is yes.

Have I mentioned that the body, psyche, and mind are not separate? They are independent parts of the whole you. The words *body, mind,* and *psyche* describe different functions, but there is no division between them. I remember teaching a corrective exercise class, at the end of which students were walking around the room, combining all of the movement and alignment techniques they had learned. One student, who said she felt taller and more comfortable than ever before, said, "It would be impossible to move this way and feel depressed at the same time." This was not merely her wishful thinking. She was feeling the actual emotional effect of good kinesthetic awareness, good alignment, relaxation, and easy movement.

Rarely are the bodily pain problems that most people have either entirely "physical" or entirely "emotional." The simple reason for this is the interconnectedness of the body, mind, and psyche. If you experience a physical injury, you will be affected mentally and emotionally, even if you suppress your awareness of it. On one level or another, your brain is aware of everything that happens in your body, which is how it regulates your bodily functions. There is a continuous sharing of information among the body, mind, and psyche.

For some people, regaining kinesthetic awareness and relaxation solves their pain problem. For others, changing tension-producing DMPs solves it. For still others, correcting their alignment is the answer. For others, acknowledging their emotions solves the problem. And for many, it is a combination of all of these that takes away the pain. These causes are not isolated from each other. Consider all of them when you are attempting to unravel the causes of your pain.

EXPLORATION 6

Lie on your back with your knees bent and your feet flat on the floor. Slowly press both of your feet into the floor, as if you were going to make a print of each foot on the floor. Notice how your pelvis tilts up off the floor. Slowly press your feet down so that your tailbone lifts about two inches off the floor, then slowly return your tailbone to the floor by reducing the pressure on your feet. The idea here is to only use your legs to make this movement happen—do not use your lower back or abdominal muscles at all. As your tailbone moves up and down, imagine that your pelvis is moving from a hinge where the sacrum connects to the bottom of the lumbar spine (see illustration 5.2 on page 85).

Does your lower back rise off the floor as your pelvis tilts up, as if they were both one piece? If so, your lower back muscles are tightening. If this is the case, repeat the movement more slowly and let your lower back sink down toward the floor as your tailbone lifts.

It might occur to you to use your abdominal muscles to keep your lower back down as your pelvis tilts up. This would work, but don't do it. By omitting the use of your abdominal muscles, you will eventually discover how to really let go of your lower back, which is the whole point of the exercise. Your lower back stays down because of gravity, not because it is being pressed down.

What is causing your pelvis to tilt up if your abdominal muscles are not involved? Observe what happens to your thighs as you press your feet into the floor. Intentionally direct your thighs and knees to move away from the hip joints as you press your feet down. This small movement of your legs away from your hips is what causes your pelvis to lift, because your pelvis is attached to your legs.

It may take a lot of slow and careful repetition before you can accomplish all of this at once. When you do, however, you will have learned how to use your legs and relax your back at the same time.

Now stand up. Remember the way your lower back felt when you were on the floor. Can you let your lower back relax when you stand, much like it did then? If not, get back on the floor and repeat the same movement a few times, and then try again. Don't give up. The floor movement is practice for learning how to stand and walk without unnecessarily tightening your lower back.

PART TWO

Exercises

7
Exercise Fundamentals

Furious activity is no substitute for understanding.
—*H. H. Williams*

THE REMAINING CHAPTERS of this book contain exercises that are designed specifically to retrain your muscles. As you do them, pay attention to the feelings of muscle effort, movement, tension, and relaxation. The more you use your kinesthetic awareness during these exercises, the better your results will be. Some of the exercises refer to a prerequisite movement exploration that is kinesthetically related to the exercise. Make sure you have done the exploration before you try the exercise.

Chapter 8 includes exercises that will help form a basis for achieving relaxation and alignment in your whole body. For this, your lumbar spine must have the appropriate curve, and your waist area muscles must support that curve when you sit, stand, and move. If your lumbar curve is not supported adequately, then other areas of your body have no choice but to compensate for that lack of support by becoming tighter and less flexible. The lumbar spine is meant to be supported by the muscles of the body center, what some people call the "core." The exercises in chapter 8 increase the muscle tone and awareness of the body center to a level where it can support the lumbar curve.

Chapters 9 through 13 include exercises specific to certain parts of the body, so if you have a pain problem in one area you can find the exercises that are most relevant. Regardless of where your pain might be, however, go through the exercises in chapter 8 first, because they will ultimately help every other part of your body. This is particularly true if you have lower back pain, because these body center exercises are all lower back exercises. If you find all of the chapter 8 exercises easy to do, then you can move on to the other chapter(s) that focus more directly on your pain problem. On the other hand, if any of these exercises are not easy, you need to practice them daily until they are.

Another important reason for going over the exercises in chapter 8 carefully is that they develop your kinesthetic sense of "lengthening your waist." In the instructions in the later chapters, I will sometimes ask you to "lengthen your waist" as you do a particular exercise. If you haven't gone through these fundamental exercises, there is a good chance that you will not know what I mean.

Creating a Long Arc

The exercises in chapter 8 are intended to give you a feeling of support in your body center, or waist, which is the area between your rib cage and your pelvis. Your lumbar spine is the back of your waist and is its main structural support. The natural curve of the lumbar spine is concave, as seen from behind (see chapter 5 for more details).

The ideal lumbar curve is as long as possible yet as curved as possible. This apparent contradiction describes the dynamic action of this part of the spine as it is moved and supported by the muscles around it. If a curved line is made as long as possible, it becomes a straight line. If a curved line is made as curved as possible, it becomes shorter. However, if the curved line is as long as possible while being as curved as possible, it becomes a long, gradual arc. That is the ideal shape for your lumbar spine.

When the lumbar spine is a long arc, the waist is as long as possible. For this to happen easily, there are a few muscular prerequisites.

First, the psoas muscles, which encourage the lumbar curve, need to be doing their job. Second, the transverse and oblique abdominal muscles need to have enough muscle tone to support the lumbar spine from the front and to lift the ribs away from the pelvis. Third, the back muscles that connect the lower back to the back of the pelvis need to relax enough to allow the pelvis to hang off the end of the lumbar spine.

Many people have a collapsed posture (flattened and/or compressed lumbar curve; see chapter 5), a posture that can cause problems throughout the rest of the body. If this is the case, the exercises in chapter 8 are essential to elongate your waist. On the other hand, if you have an exaggerated lumbar curve, these exercises will teach your back muscles to relax and lengthen.

Depending on your habitual posture and use of your waist muscles, you may find some of the exercises in chapter 8 more relevant than others. In general, if you are following the instructions carefully, moving slowly, and finding an exercise easy, then you are probably doing it correctly. The goal of practicing these exercises is for them to become so easy that you will automatically use your muscles and spine this way throughout the day.

Doing All Exercises Slowly and with Full Awareness

The more slowly you do the exercises, the more benefit you will receive from them. Moving slowly will allow you to pay more attention to what you are doing. It also presents more of a challenge to your muscles. If you are accustomed to doing other types of exercises quickly, then you may need to remind yourself frequently to slow down as you are learning the exercises from this book. I often tell people that if they only have ten minutes to do these exercises, they are better off doing two or three of them slowly and mindfully, rather than attempting to cram as many exercises as possible into the ten minutes. More is not necessarily better—aim for quality, not quantity.

A Word Regarding Painful Exercise

The exercises in this book are not intended to be painful. If you are in pain while doing an exercise, it is likely that you will not be able to relax, which will undermine the purpose of the exercise. Also, pain is usually an indicator that you are either doing the exercise too forcefully or too fast, or that your body is just not ready to do it. If you feel pain while doing any of these exercises, respect your body, be patient, and back off a little. If the pain is such that you can let it be there and still relax around it, then you can proceed slowly. If the pain is such that you cannot relax, then modify the exercise or don't do it.

For years I resisted using the term *exercises* to refer to these corrective movements and positions, because for many people, the word *exercise* means working through pain, pushing hard, and straining muscles. None of these concepts apply to these movements. On the other hand, the term *exercise* also suggests something that you can practice—which definitely applies to these movements. So for lack of a better word, I refer to these movements and positions as exercises.

8

Lower Back Pain, Part I

EXERCISE 1: LUMBAR CURVE AND FLATTEN

Prerequisite

Exploration 1 (see page 9)

Objective

The exaggerated waist flexion and extension in this exercise improves the tone of the waist muscles.

Position

- Lie on your back with your knees bent and your feet flat on the floor. Your legs and feet should be parallel to each other. Place your hands under your head.
- Using your abdominal muscles, press your lower back into the floor. The curve of your lower back will flatten, and your tailbone will lift slightly off the floor. At the same time, use the same abdominal muscles, along with your arms, to lift your head and upper chest. Point your elbows up. Your shoulders will lift off the floor.

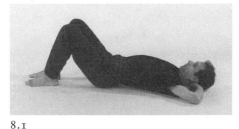
8.1

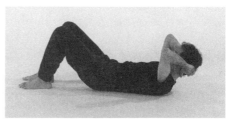
8.2

- Next, reverse the motion by releasing your abdominal muscles and engaging your lower back muscles. This will exaggerate the lumbar curve and press your tailbone into the floor. As you do this, slowly lower your head back to the floor and let your arms relax completely.
- Continue moving slowly, back and forth, exhaling when you flatten the lumbar curve and inhaling as you increase it.
- Repeat the entire exercise slowly 15 times.

Sensing

Feel how your abdominal and lower back muscles work as partners in this movement. Notice that when your abdominals engage, your back muscles release, and vice versa.

Imagining

Imagine that your pelvis is a ball, rolling down toward your feet, then up toward your head.

EXERCISE 2: PELVIS LIFT WITH LEGS

Prerequisite

Exploration 6 (see page 135)

Objective

The pelvis should be able to make a small movement that is independent of the lumbar spine. This exercise asks the lower back muscles to let go of the pelvis and the hip muscles to let go of the legs. This exercise is the same as exploration 6.

Position

- Lie on your back with your knees bent and your feet flat on the floor. Your legs should be parallel to each other. Place your arms on the floor and your hands on your abdomen.
- Slowly press both of your feet into the floor, as if you were going to make a print of each foot on the floor. Allow your thighs to

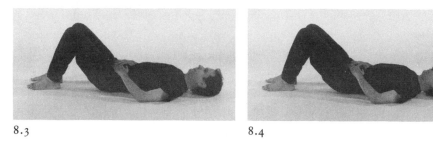

8.3   8.4

slide slightly toward your knees, as if each thigh were being pulled away from its hip socket. This small movement of your legs will lift your pelvis so your tailbone is about two inches off the floor. Relax your abdominal muscles *completely*—do *not* use them to tilt your pelvis. Keep your lower back relaxed, so it *remains on the floor,* even as your pelvis tilts upward. The muscular effort for this motion is coming only from your legs. If your lower spine lifts off the floor, you are either (1) not releasing your back muscles or (2) lifting your pelvis too high.

- For some people this is very easy, and there is no need to practice it further. However, if it seems difficult or impossible—which it might—practice this exercise every day until the coordination of movements becomes automatic (it eventually will). This is a small, subtle movement.
- Repeat this motion very slowly 20 times.

Sensing

Feel how your lower back remains on the floor because you have allowed it to relax, *not* because you have pushed it down with your abdominal muscles.

Imagining

Imagine there is a hinge between your pelvis and your last lumbar vertebra—the pelvis part of the hinge moves and the vertebra does not. Imagine that your knees are hanging over a bar; as you press your feet down, the bar gently pulls diagonally and upward away from your hips, in the same direction that your thighs are pointing.

Note: As your sense of this movement becomes clear, you will eventually be able to sense the same relaxation in your lower back even when you are standing up.

EXERCISE 3: ABDOMINAL PULL-IN

Prerequisites
Explorations 2 (see page 29) and 3 (see page 51)

Objective
This simple exercise begins to train your abdominal muscles to support your lumbar spine from the front.

Position
- Lie on your back with your knees bent and your feet flat on the floor. Place your arms on the floor and your hands on your abdomen.
- As you exhale, slowly lift both feet about 5 inches off the floor, keeping your knees bent. Inhale. On your next exhalation, slowly return your feet to the floor. As you raise and lower your legs, use your abdominal muscles to keep your pelvis still and to press your lower back into the floor. Even though you are engaging your abdominal muscles, *do not shorten the distance between your pubic bone and the front of your chest.* Relax your abdominal muscles completely when your feet return to the floor.
- Repeat slowly as many times as possible, gradually working up to 15 repetitions.

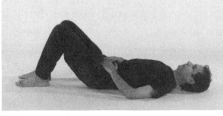
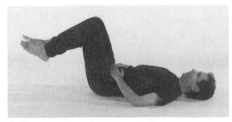

8.5   8.6

Sensing

Sense how your pelvis and lower spine are stabilized by engaging your abdominal muscles.

Imagining

Imagine that your lumbar spine is cemented to the floor as you raise and lower your legs.

Note: This exercise and a few others involves flattening your lower back. The purpose of this is *not* to eliminate the essential lumbar curve. That will not happen from doing these exercises. We are using the flattening as a way to help you sense how the muscles in the front of your waist affect your lower back.

EXERCISE 4: Psoas Release and Lengthen

Prerequisites

Explorations 1 (see page 9), 2 (see page 29), 3 (see page 51), and 6 (see page 135)

Objective

This exercise encourages the psoas muscles to stay relaxed and long (see chapter 5 for details about the psoas muscles).

Position

- Lie on your back with your knees bent and your feet flat on the floor.
- Raise your right knee to your chest and hold your right leg with

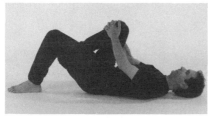 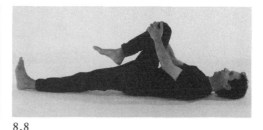

8.7   8.8

your hands. As you do this, make sure that your pelvis remains in the same position on the floor.

- Next, slowly straighten your left leg along the floor. Again, make sure that your pelvis remains in the same position. There will be a tendency for your lower back to rise off the floor as your left leg straightens. Relax your back muscles, and keep your lower back and pelvis in the same position throughout the exercise. If you are unable to straighten your leg completely without tilting your pelvis, stop at the point where your lower back raises off the floor.
- Slowly reverse the movement of your left leg, by bending your knee and sliding your heel along the floor. Return your left leg to the starting position.
- Repeat the same movement 10 times, then reverse legs and repeat the movement with your right leg.

Sensing

Feel how the movement of each leg is controlled by the psoas muscle at the top of the thigh, not by the muscles around the knee.

Imagining

Imagine that your abdomen is sinking into your lower back, while your lower back lengthens as you slowly move your leg back and forth.

EXERCISE 5: LENGTHENING THE WAIST: WALL SLIDE

Prerequisites

Explorations 1 (see page 9), 2 (see page 29), 3 (see page 51), and 6 (see page 135)

Objective

This exercise will give you an exaggerated sense of how the action of your abdominal muscles can lengthen your waist vertically. A longer waist means less compression on your lower back.

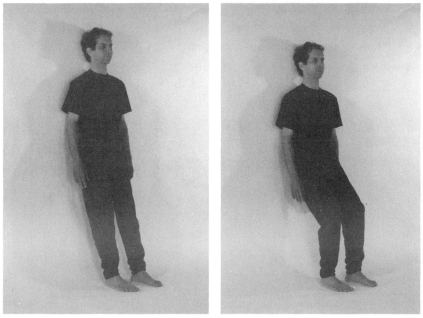

8.9   8.10

Position

- Stand with your legs straight and your back leaning against the wall. Your feet should be parallel to each other, hip-width apart, and about 12 to 15 inches away from the wall. Relax and let the wall hold you up. Look directly in front of you, with your head level and touching the wall. If your head does not rest comfortably against the wall, place a folded towel between the back of your head and the wall.
- First, bend your knees so that you slide down the wall about 6 inches. In the bent-knee position, use your abdominal muscles to press your lumbar spine toward the wall (there should be very little space between your lower back and the wall). Do not engage your buttock muscles at all. *Do not shorten the distance between your pubic bone and the front of your chest.* If your chest pulls forward or down as you press your back toward the

wall, you are overusing your rectus abdominal muscles (shortening your waist in the front).

- Next, slowly straighten your knees and slide back up the wall. As you do this, keep your abdominal muscles engaged and your lower back pressed toward the wall as much as possible. When you return to the starting position, you will notice that you have lengthened your waist without tightening your back muscles.
- Slide slowly down and up 15 times.

Sensing

Sense how your abdominal muscles are causing two different actions: (1) the lower abdominals are pressing your lower back toward the wall, and (2) the upper abdominals are lifting your ribs. The result is a longer waist. Sense also that your lower back muscles do not need to engage in order to accomplish this.

Imagining

When you are in the bent-knee position, imagine that your pelvis is a level bucket that is full of water. As you are sliding up the wall, imagine that the bucket remains level so the water does not spill over the front.

Note: This exercise requires that your abdominal muscles exaggerate the action they normally make while you're standing. I am not suggesting that you should forcefully suck in your gut all day long. Many people have abandoned the muscles that are used in this exercise, so their posture is collapsed. In the standing position, this abdominal action would ideally be an automatic function of muscle tone. Until you reach that point, practice this exaggeration. Gradually, you will be able to get the feeling of a long waist when you are standing (without a wall). As your back relaxes and your abdominal muscles wake up, your muscles will do this automatically. If your breathing becomes difficult during this exercise, your back muscles are so tight that the sides and back of your ribs are not moving when you breathe. In this case, use less effort in your abdominal muscles, go more slowly, and focus on relaxing your back.

9

Lower Back Pain, Part II

EXERCISE 6: WALL SUPINE HIP FLEXION

Prerequisite

Exploration 1 (see page 9)

Objective

This position lengthens the posterior leg and hip muscles. It is also useful in restoring a flattened lumbar curve to its natural shape. The muscles of the backs of the hips and thighs attach the legs to the pelvis. When these muscles are tight, they pull down on the back of the pelvis. If they are constantly tight, there will be a flattening effect on the lumbar spine and its discs.

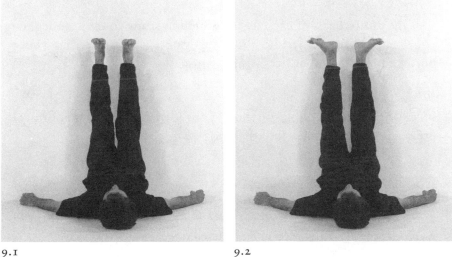

9.1   9.2

Position, Part 1

- Lie on your back, with your arms outstretched and your legs flat against the wall. You feet should be parallel, hip-width apart. Your knees should be straight and the bottom of your pelvis as close to the wall as possible.
- Let your lower back sink into the floor. If you cannot get the bottom of your pelvis (sit bones) flat against the wall, then position your pelvis far enough away from the wall that you are able to straighten your knees. Over time, as your leg muscles loosen, move in closer to the wall.
- While in this position, intermittently flex and relax your feet.
- Stay in this position for up to 3 minutes.

Position, Part 2

- Lie on your back, with your arms outstretched and your legs flat against the wall. Your knees should be straight and your feet parallel, hip-width apart. Position the bottom of your pelvis (sit bones) as close to the wall as possible.
- Using your buttock muscles, turn both legs and feet outward, keeping your heels close to each other. Hold this position for 5 seconds, then return to the starting position.
- Repeat slowly 20 times.

Sensing

Feel the entire back of each leg lengthening from your sit bones to your heels. In part 2, feel how turning your legs is initiated by your buttock muscles and not your thigh muscles.

Imagining

Imagine there is a sandbag on top of your lower abdomen that firmly presses your lower back into the floor.

EXERCISE 7: SIDE RELEASE

Prerequisites

Explorations 4 (see page 73) and 5 (see page 106)

Objective

This exercise lengthens the sides of the waist, which benefits the shoulders and hips as well as the lower back.

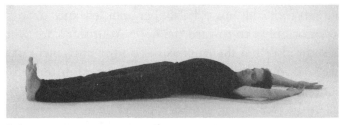

9.3

Position

- Lie on your back with your legs extended straight and your arms on the floor above your shoulders.
- Begin by lengthening the right side of your waist, extending your right arm and right leg to form a lengthening straight line. Relax.
- Next, lengthen the left side of your waist by extending your left arm and left leg to form a lengthening straight line. Relax.
- Alternate slowly, extending one side, then the other. Keep your neck completely relaxed, so that your head rolls from side to side as your arms and legs extend. Do not arch your lower back off the floor; use your side muscles, not your back muscles, to do this movement.
- Repeat 6 times on each side.

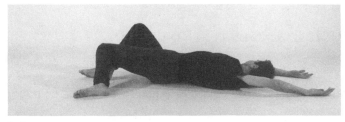

9.4

Optional Position

- Lie on your back with both knees bent and your feet flat on the floor. Your feet should be at least 12 inches apart, and your arms should be relaxed on the floor above your shoulders.
- Begin by dropping your left knee in toward your right leg, so your left foot rolls inward also. Let your left knee drop as far as it comfortably can toward the floor. Your left knee will fall to the right also, but the emphasis is on the movement of the left knee. As you do this, lengthen the muscles on the left side of your waist, so your left pelvis is pulled along with your left leg. At the same time, extend your left arm along the floor in a straight line away from your left knee. Your entire left side is lengthened from your knee to your hand. *Relax your lower back muscles* as you do this. Let your neck relax also, so that your head rolls a little.
- Return to the original position, then do the same movement with your right leg, hip, waist, and arm.
- Alternate slowly from one side to the other 6 times.

Sensing

Feel your leg and arm result from lengthening of the entire side of your torso. Sense also how the lengthening of one side is caused by the active shortening of the opposite side. Because of this, little effort is needed to extend your limbs.

Imagining

Imagine how your spine is bending into opposite sideways curves as you lengthen and shorten the sides of your waist.

EXERCISE 8: CENTER ROTATION

Prerequisites

Explorations 1 (see page 9), 4 (see page 73), and 5 (see page 106)

Objective

This exercise will restore your kinesthetic sense of waist rotation while releasing your lower back muscles. This exercise is the same as exploration 5.

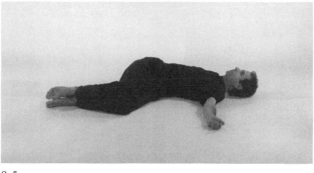

9.5

Position, Part 1: Lower Body

- Lie on your back with your knees bent and your feet flat on the floor next to each other. Place your arms on the floor.
- Drop both of your knees to the left so that your pelvis rotates to the left.
- Engage your abdominal oblique muscles to slowly roll your pelvis and legs up across the midline and over to the right. Continue the movement until your knees have dropped to the right. Reverse the movement again, using your abdominal obliques to slowly move your pelvis and legs back to the midline, then dropping your knees to the left.
- Continue slowly moving your pelvis and legs back and forth from right to left. *Do not engage your back muscles.* Initiate the movement from your abdominal obliques, not your leg muscles. This means that your pelvis moves first and your legs follow. Use your leg muscles as little as possible as your legs move from side to side.
- Repeat 6 times to each side.

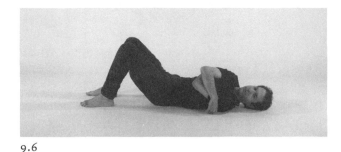

9.6

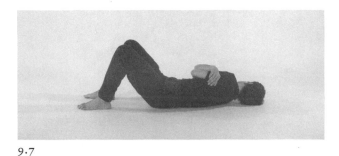

9.7

Position, Part 2: Upper Body

- Lie on your back with your knees bent and your feet flat on the floor, hip-width apart. Cross your arms over your chest so your hands are hanging down on either side of your chest.
- Slowly roll your chest to the left as far as you can. As in the previous exercise, the goal is to isolate your abdominal oblique muscles, but this time you're turning your chest.
- Next, rotate your chest to the right. Continue rolling back and forth.
- Remember that you are rolling, not lifting your back off the ground. Your head should stay in contact with the ground. Do not move your pelvis, keep your lumbar spine rooted to the floor, and do not engage any muscles along your spine. Completely relax your shoulders, arms, and neck, so they are carried by the movement of your waist. Your head will roll a little from side to side, not because you are engaging your neck muscles but because it is pulled by the turning of your spine.
- Repeat slowly 6 times to each side.

Sensing

Feel how your body center can initiate and control the movement of your pelvis and upper body.

Imagining

Imagine you are a floppy puppet that can move using only your abdominal muscles.

EXERCISE 9: DOUBLE LEG SLIDE AND LIFT

Prerequisites

Explorations 1 (see page 9), 2 (see page 29), and 3 (see page 51)

Objective

This exercise develops the psoas muscles to stabilize the lower back. You should master the previous exercise before attempting this one.

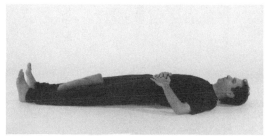

9.8

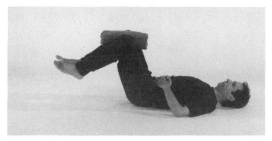

9.9

Position

- Lie on your back with your legs extended out straight. Place a rolled towel (about 5 inches thick) between your knees. Place your arms on the floor and your hands on your abdomen.
- Slowly bend both knees. Keep them pointing straight up, and let your heels drag on the floor. Keep the towel between your knees by pressing them together. Relax your ankles. When your feet are close to your buttocks, continue the movement by slowly lifting both feet about 5 inches off the floor. Then reverse the movement by sliding your feet slowly back to the starting position. Keep your lower back long and pressed into the floor while you do this.
- Repeat up to 30 times.

Sensing

Feel how your leg movement is controlled by your psoas muscles, and your lumbar spine is kept long by using your abdominal muscles.

Imagining

Imagine that your legs are being moved up and down by a string that is suspended from the ceiling and looped around each knee.

IO

Hip, Knee, and Leg Pain

EXERCISE 10: LATERAL HIP ROTATION

Prerequisites

Explorations 4 (see page 73) and 5 (see page 106)

Objective

This exercise activates and releases the outer thigh and hip muscles that control the alignment of the pelvis, legs, and knees.

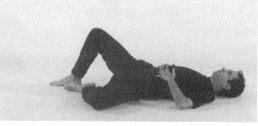

10.1

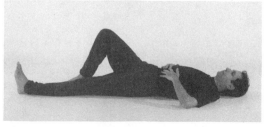

10.2

Position

- Lie on your back with your knees bent and your feet flat on the floor, hip-width apart. Place your arms on the floor and your hands on your abdomen. Then drop your left knee outward so the outside of your foot is against the floor.
- Begin by sliding your left foot forward along the floor, with the sole parallel to your right leg. Your knee will gradually straighten. As you do this, try to keep the outside of your left foot against the floor; you will feel the muscles engage in the back of your left hip to keep your left leg turned out. When your knee is fully straightened, rotate your leg to neutral position (with your toes pointing straight up) and pause for a few seconds.
- Then turn your left leg outward again, begin bending your left knee, and slowly return to the starting position. There is no need to hold your pelvis still as you bend and straighten your leg—it's okay if it rolls from side to side.
- Slowly repeat this movement 10 times.
- Reverse legs, and repeat the same movement with the right leg.

Sensing

Feel how the control of your leg rotation and your knee/foot alignment comes primarily from the muscles in your buttocks, not from those in your thighs.

Imagining

Visualize the lateral rotation of your thighbone, which is like a long axle being rotated between the hip and the knee. Visualize how this rotation affects the position of your knee.

EXERCISE 11: LATERAL LEG LENGTHENER

Prerequisites

Explorations 4 (see page 73) and 5 (see page 106)

Objective

This exercise lengthens the side and posterior hip muscles by turning the leg inward.

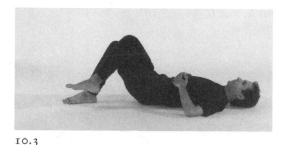

10.3

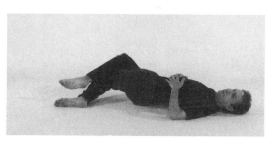

10.4

Position

- Lie on your back with your knees bent and your feet flat on the floor, hip-width apart. Place your arms on the floor and your hands on your abdomen. Then cross your right knee over your left knee. Your left foot remains on the floor; your right foot does not.
- Drop your knees to the right. Use the weight of your right leg to help move the left toward the floor. Next, engage the muscles on the inside of your left thigh to press your left knee farther toward the floor. Hold this position for 5 seconds, then relax your leg muscles completely for five seconds, keeping your knees dropped to the right. Throughout the movement, keep your upper back flat and your shoulders on the floor.

- Repeat the same procedure of engaging and relaxing the left thigh muscles for a total of 6 repetitions, with 5 seconds engaged and 5 seconds relaxed for each repetition. Return the legs to the starting position after the last repetition.
- Reverse legs and repeat the same movements, this time dropping your knees to the left. Repeat 6 times.

Sensing

Feel the muscles on the inside of your thigh help to rotate your leg inward; the more this happens, the more you will feel the muscles stretch in the side of your hip and your buttocks. Also, if you are able to keep your upper back and shoulders flat on the floor, feel how your spine twists all the way up to your neck. This twist is a good stretch for your entire spine.

Imagining

Visualize how your waist twists, like a wet cloth twists when it is being wrung out.

EXERCISE 12: KNEE BEND

Prerequisites

Explorations 1 (see page 9) and 6 (see page 135)

Objective

This exercise retrains the leg muscles to take much of the load off the back when standing and bending.

Position

- Stand facing the edge of a door, with your feet parallel and near the end of the door. Hold on to the doorknobs.
- Slowly bend your knees until your knees and hips form a 90-degree angle. As you bend down, press your weight into the heels of your feet as much as possible. Keep your torso vertical (do not lean backward). Keep your knees over your ankles the

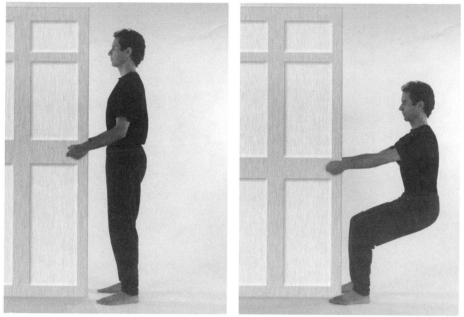

10.5   10.6

entire time; your lower legs will remain in the same position (perpendicular to the floor) throughout the movement.

- When you reach the 90-degree angle (or as close to it as you can comfortably get), stay there for 15 seconds, continuing to press your heels into the floor. Then slowly return to the starting position, remembering to press your heels down, keep your torso vertical, and keep your lower legs stationary.
- Repeat the cycle 6 times.

Sensing

Feel how your legs, not your lower back, do the work of getting you up and down.

Imagining

Imagine that your legs are rooted to the ground like a tree while you are standing.

II

Upper Back, Shoulder, and Neck Pain

EXERCISE 13: STANDING HIP FLEXION/FORWARD BEND

Prerequisites

Explorations 1 (see page 9), 2 (see page 29), 3 (see page 51), and 6 (see page 135)

Objective

This exercise has two parts. The purpose of the first is to develop a sense of lengthening in the entire back of the body, while at the same time using the back muscles. The purpose of the second is to relax the entire back of the body.

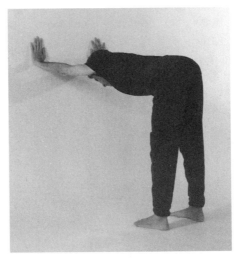

II.I

Position, Part 1: Standing Hip Flexion

- Stand with your feet about hip-width apart, about 3 feet away from a wall. Bend forward from your hip joints, keeping your entire torso long and straight; place your hands on the wall in front of you. Your knees should be straight, not hyperextended. Place your hands as low on the wall as possible while still bending *at the hips*. Do not bend at your waist. If you are unable to keep your lumbar spine straight, move your hands up the wall until you can. This is where you should place your hands when you begin practicing this exercise. Adjust your feet so they are directly under your pelvis and still parallel.

- While in this position, maintain a long waist and keep your heels on the floor. This is an active position; use your abdominal muscles to support and lengthen your waist and to keep the natural lumbar curve. As your back muscles lengthen in this position, you may be able to walk your hands a bit lower down the wall. Over time, you will be able to get your hips to bend at a right angle in this exercise, so that your back is parallel to the floor.

- Remain in this position for 30 seconds, eventually increasing to 2 minutes. To come out of this position, step one leg forward and walk your hands up the wall.

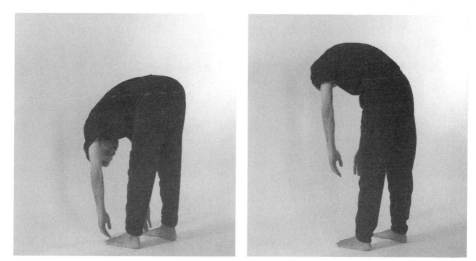

11.2   11.3

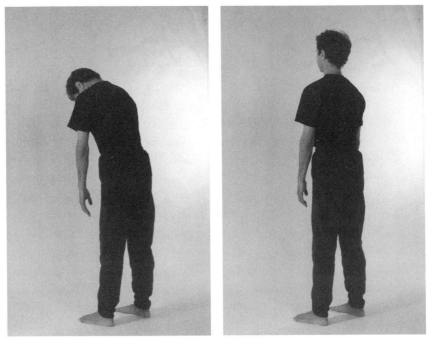

11.4   11.5

Position, Part 2: Forward Bend

- Stand with your feet hip-width apart and parallel. Relax your torso and neck so your head hangs down. Note that you're hanging from your hips and not your waist. Keep your knees straight but not hyperextended.
- Hang in this position with your arms relaxed. Breathe. Relax your neck. Stay in this position for up to 1 minute.
- To exit this position, slowly come up by pressing your heels into the ground, rolling your pelvis backward, and "stacking" your vertebrae from the bottom up. Keep your knees straight (unless you have lower back pain, in which case, bend them comfortably). Relax your back muscles as much as possible, and pull your abdominal muscles in and up, as if you are pushing yourself up the front. Keep your neck, shoulders, and arms relaxed the entire time. The last part of you to come up is your head.

Sensing, Part 1: Standing Hip Flexion

Feel your waist lengthening continuously, as if the bottom of your pelvis and the top of your head were reaching in opposite directions. In addition, feel your legs lengthening from your sit bones to your heels.

Imagining, Part 1: Standing Hip Flexion

Imagine that your hands are stuck to the wall. At the same time, picture a horizontal bar directly in front of your hip joints. Imagine that the bar is being pulled diagonally up and back, so that you are being stretched away from the wall by the bar. You may feel a stretch in your shoulders as well.

Sensing, Part 2: Forward Bend

As you are hanging down, sense how the weight of your head lengthens your neck and upper back muscles.

Imagining, Part 2: Forward Bend

Imagine that you have the upper body of a rag doll. As you come up, imagine a hand pushing up against the front of your spine, inch by inch, gradually bringing you to a standing position.

EXERCISE 14: WALL PUSH-UP

Prerequisites

Explorations 2 (see page 29) and 6 (see page 135)

Objective

This exercise activates the upper back muscles and opens the chest while lengthening the spine.

Position

- Stand facing a wall, with your feet hip-width apart about 15 inches away from it. Keep your feet hip-width apart and parallel. Place your hands on the wall at shoulder height, with your fingers pointing diagonally inward and your elbows straight.

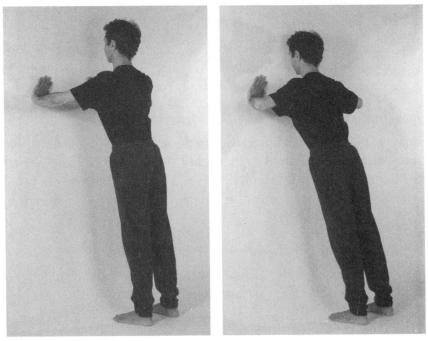

11.6   11.7

- Slowly lean your entire body forward, bending your elbows as you lower yourself closer to the wall. Keep your entire body straight and your feet firmly on the ground. Keep your neck in line with the rest of your spine. Relax your arms, shoulders, and neck as much as possible, so you are not tensing any unnecessary muscles in order to do the movement. Continue until your nose is a few inches from the wall, then reverse directions and return to the starting position. As you move away from the wall, keep your chest open and wide.
- Repeat very slowly 10 times.

Sensing

Sense that you are using the leverage of the bones in your arms to move your body, rather than using only muscle strength (as in a conventional push-up).

Imagining

Imagine that your hands are glued to the wall and your feet are glued to the ground as you do this exercise.

EXERCISE 15: TORSO ROTATION WITH ARM CIRCLE

Prerequisites

Explorations 1 (see page 9), 3 (see page 51), and 4 (see page 73)

Objective

The goal here is to sense how arm movement is supported by movement of the torso and how this support helps the shoulder to relax.

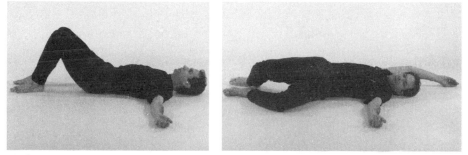

11.8   11.9

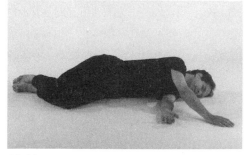 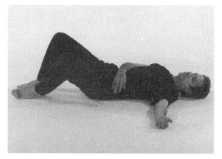

11.10   11.11

Position

- Lie on your back with your knees bent and your feet flat on the floor and close together. Place your left arm straight out at your side, and place your right arm along side of your body.
- Begin the movement by slowly dragging your right arm along the floor, away from your right leg and toward your head. As your arm moves upward, actively lengthen the right side of your torso. As your arm gets near your head, drop both knees to the left, and use your abdominal muscles to roll over onto your left side. Your right arm will follow the movement of your torso, not lead it. Continue making a circle with your right arm, dragging it above your head and around to your left side as your body rolls. Bring your right hand over your left and continue the circle so your hand crosses over your waist. As your arm crosses back to your right side, roll onto your back again and return your legs to the vertical starting position. Your arm has made one complete circle.
- Keep your neck completely relaxed throughout this entire movement. Let your head roll as a consequence of your torso's movement, but do not pick up your head. For neck comfort, you can place a pillow under your head, as long as the pillow is not so high that it interferes with the rolling of your head.
- If moving your arm above the shoulder causes pain, do not continue with that part of the circle. Instead, stop dragging your arm at the point where the shoulder pain begins, and start rolling onto your side. In this case, your arm will move in a long arc in the air, over your chest, from right to left, eventually landing on the floor as you roll onto your left side. Do your best to feel that your arm is moving as a part of your torso, a movement that is initiated in your abdominal muscles.
- Repeat 6 times, then reverse arms and the direction of the movement.

Sensing

Feel how lengthening the side of your torso allows your arm to reach farther above your head, which in turn makes it almost effortless to roll onto your side. Feel how the entire movement is smooth and continuous. Sense the heaviness of your arm, and only use the arm muscles that are absolutely necessary to complete the circle.

Imagining

Imagine that you were doing this exercise on a sandy beach and you can see the big circle around your upper body that is made by your hand dragging along the sand. For your hand to stay in the sand, your shoulder needs to stay relaxed.

EXERCISE 16: NECK ROLLS

Prerequisites

Explorations 4 (see page 73) and 5 (see page 106)

Objective

This movement releases habitual tension from the neck.

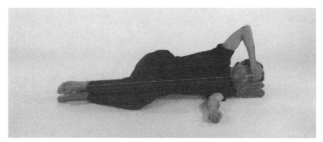

11.12

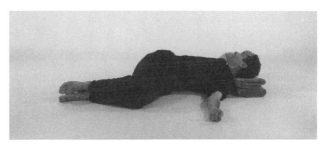

11.13

Position

- Lie on your left side. Place a folded towel or a pillow under your head so that your neck is comfortable. Bend your hips and knees at 90-degree angles. Place your left arm on the floor, pointing straight out in front of you, with your right hand on your forehead.
- Using your right hand, slowly roll your head to the right as far as it will comfortably go, then roll it back to the starting position.
- Continue to roll your head right and left slowly. Do *not* use your neck muscles to move your head—*relax your neck*. Use only your right arm and hand to move your head. Let your chest open and your torso twist as your head is able to turn farther.
- Continue rolling your head for 1 to 2 minutes, then turn onto your right side and repeat the same procedure.

Sensing

Feel how the range of motion in your neck depends on the ability of your chest and abdomen to lengthen and stretch. Feel how your head moves more smoothly when you let your hand move it than when you use your neck muscles to do so.

Imagining

Imagine that your head is a ball, rolling smoothly from side to side.

12

Shoulder, Elbow, and Wrist Pain

EXERCISE 17: UPPER BACK FLEX AND EXTEND

Prerequisite

Exploration 1 (see page 9)

Objective

These positions activate muscles in the back and shoulders that are needed for good shoulder alignment.

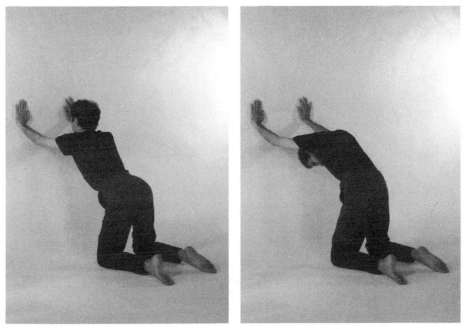

12.1   12.2

Position

- Kneel on the floor with your knees hip-width apart about 15 inches from a wall. Place your hands against the wall and above your head. Your hips should be bent at almost 90 degrees. Let your back arch.
- Slowly pull your shoulder blades diagonally inward, as if you were aiming them toward your tailbone. As you do this, increase the arch in your lower back. Maintain this position for 5 seconds.
- Next, let your head drop forward, and curve your upper back so it has a humped shape. Maintain this position for 5 seconds.
- Alternate slowly between the two positions. Repeat a total of 10 times.

Sensing

Feel how the muscles between and below your shoulder blades increase the arch in your back and pull your shoulder blades down.

Imagining

Picture how your entire spine is curving one way and then the other as you make the movements.

EXERCISE 18: LATERAL SHOULDER ROTATION

Prerequisite

Exploration 1 (see page 9)

Objective

This movement opens the chest and activates the muscles connecting the back to the arms.

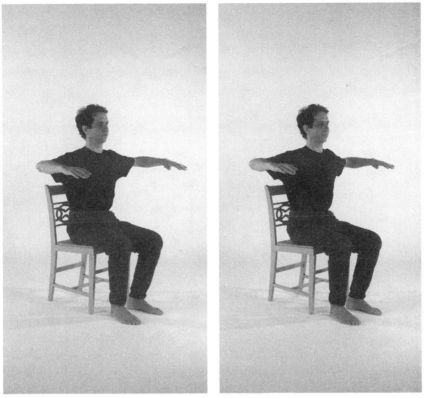

12.3   12.4

Position, Part 1

- Sit on the front half of a chair, so you are resting on your sit bones. Hold your arms a little below your shoulders, with the upper arms pointing out to the left and right sides, elbows bent at 90 degrees, and palms facing downward.
- Slowly pull your upper arms diagonally backward and down as far as comfortably possible, by squeezing your shoulder blades together. You will feel the muscles between and below your shoulder blades engage. Maintain this position for 5 seconds. Keep your waist as long possible. Return your arms to the starting position and pause for a few seconds.
- Repeat a total of 10 times.

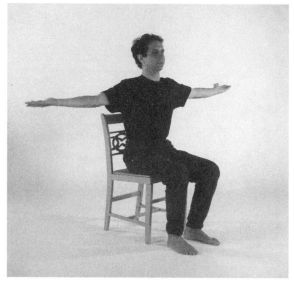

12.5

Position, Part 2

- Sit on the front half of a chair, so you are resting on your sit bones. Hold your arms straight out to the sides at shoulder height, with your palms facing forward.
- Slowly rotate both arms backward, so that your palms turn up and continue turning behind you. Rotate them as far as you comfortably can. Then pull your arms backward by squeezing your shoulder blades together. Maintain this position for 10 seconds.
- Relax completely, then repeat for a total of 5 repetitions.

Sensing

Feel how the rotation of your arms comes from the muscles between and below your shoulder blades, as well as from the arms themselves.

Imagining

Imagine that your arms are wings that begin along either side of your spine. Picture your wings pulling back when you move your arms back.

EXERCISE 19: SEATED SHOULDER RELEASE

Prerequisite

Exploration 1 (see page 9)

Objective

This exercise lengthens and widens the upper back, while releasing the arms from tense back muscles.

Position

- Sit on the front half of a chair, so you are resting on your sit bones. Bend your elbows and place your hands on top of each other, with palms on your abdomen.
- Relax your neck so that your head drops forward. Let your chest cave in as you bring your right elbow forward, bending your right wrist, and keeping your right palm pressed to your abdomen. Let your torso rotate a few inches to the left. Feel

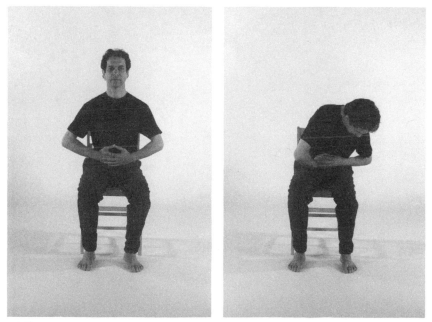

12.6   12.7

your shoulder blades moving apart and your upper back lengthening and widening. *Relax your neck.* Maintain this position for 10 to 15 seconds.

- Sit upright again. Take a slow, full breath.
- Repeat 6 times, then do the same movement 6 times using the left arm. Remember to sit upright and pause between each forward bend.

Sensing

Feel how the caving in of your chest causes your upper back to widen more, and how the more your upper back widens, the farther forward you can move your elbow.

Imagining

Picture your shoulder blades gliding freely over the back of your ribs.

13

Resting, Standing, Sitting, Walking

THESE EXERCISES are aimed specifically at making the everyday activities of resting, standing, sitting, and walking more comfortable. They are intended to be incorporated into these activities so that eventually the activities themselves become "exercises."

Resting

Resting in a position that releases muscular strain and tension can be a relief, as well as a way to gradually retrain muscles to relax. Here is a rest position that relaxes the entire back. In particular, it can relieve pain in your lower back by encouraging the psoas muscles to release.

EXERCISE 20: LUMBAR RELAXATION

Position
- Lie on your back with your lower legs supported on a chair seat or low table, so that your hips and knees are bent at about 90 degrees. Let your legs relax completely. Ideally, your legs should remain parallel to each other when they relax in this position. If your knees fall far out to the sides, you can tie a scarf or rope in a loop around your legs, just above the knees. This will allow you to relax your legs completely while still keeping them parallel.

- If your lower back resists resting flat on the floor in this position and/or feels painfully unsupported, try placing a rolled towel (about 2 to 3 inches thick) under the lumbar curve. If the towel makes you more comfortable, keep it there. If it makes you more uncomfortable, don't use it.
- Another option is to place a rolled towel (about 2 to 3 inches thick) under the curve of your neck to help reinforce the natural curve of your neck. The towel is not under your head—only your neck. Again, only use this suggestion if it increases your comfort.
- Relax in this position for 5 to 15 minutes.

Sensing

Feel your lower back sinking into the floor as it relaxes.

Imagining

Imagine your spine lengthening as if your head and your tailbone were being pulled in opposite directions.

Standing

If the previous exercises in this book were easy for you, then comfortable standing with good alignment will be as well. The most important point to remember is to keep your waist long—do not collapse your waist. As mentioned earlier, this requires that (1) your psoas muscles have made your lumbar curve a long arc; (2) your abdominal muscle tone supports your lumbar spine from the front, sides, and back; and (3) your back muscles are as long and relaxed as possible.

Often, people who have a caved-in chest try to stand up taller by pulling their shoulders back. This does not work, because it is the spine itself that keeps the upper body upright, not the shoulders. When you are standing, let your shoulders and arms relax. Let your head float up, without tightening your shoulders. Sense the whole back of your body getting longer, from the back of your head to your heels.

Here are two simple exercises that will help with standing.

EXERCISE 21: Standing

Prerequisites

Explorations 2 (see page 29), 3 (see page 51), and 6 (see page 135)

Objective

This position encourages the lengthening of all the muscles in the back of the body, allowing you to stand with better alignment.

Position

- Stand with the front half of your feet on a phone book, 2 to 3 inches high. Place your heels firmly on the ground.
- Center most of your weight on your heels. Keep your pelvis *under* your torso (not pushed out in front of it), use your abdominal muscles to lengthen your waist, relax your neck, shoulders, and arms and look straight ahead. Tilt your entire body slightly forward, without lifting your heels.
- Remain in this position for 1 to 2 minutes.

Sensing

Sense how the distance between your pelvis and ribs gets longer.

Imagining

Imagine that your head is floating up toward the sky and your heels are extending down into the ground, so that the entire back of your body is getting longer in both directions.

EXERCISE 22: Standing Shoulder Blade Rolls

Prerequisites

Explorations 2 (see page 29), 3 (see page 51), and 6 (see page 135)

Objective

This simple exercise activates the shoulder and back muscles that help remind the upper spine to lengthen.

Position

- Stand with the front half of your feet on a phone book, 2 to 3 inches high. Place your heels firmly on the ground.
- First, raise your shoulders up toward your ears, then slowly roll your shoulders back by using your upper back muscles to pull your shoulder blades together. While continuing to pull your shoulders back, also pull them down. Your arms should remain relaxed at your sides. Feel how your thoracic spine (the part behind your chest) is pressed forward by this action of your back muscles. Keep your neck relaxed and your lower back long. Maintain this position for 10 seconds. Then completely relax your shoulders and arms, but keep your spine long and your head up.
- Repeat 3 times.

Sensing

Feel how your shoulder blade muscles help to open your chest. When your chest is open, notice how your shoulders and arms can completely relax without the chest collapsing.

Imagining

As in the previous exercise, imagine that your head is floating up toward the sky and your heels are extending down into the ground, so that the entire back of your body is getting longer in both directions.

Sitting

Sitting is much like standing, except that your weight is supported by your pelvis instead of your feet. Ideally, your weight should be balanced evenly over your sit bones (see chapter 5) so that your pelvis is centered in a neutral alignment. If your psoas muscles stop doing their job while you are sitting in a chair, your pelvis will roll backward and your weight will land behind your sit bones. This position may feel comfortable to your back because your psoas and back muscles are taking a vacation. However, in the long run, this collapsed posture will distort your natural lumbar curve and injure the lumbar discs.

You can use the back of your chair to help keep you balanced on your sit bones if you sit with the back of your pelvis right up against the back of the chair. Sitting in a chair that puts your knees higher than your hips (such as a car with bucket seats) will cause your pelvis to roll backward into the collapsed posture. In this case, if you place a folded towel under your pelvis to make your hips level with your knees, you will notice immediately that it is easier for you to sit tall. Some people also find it very helpful to use a rolled-up towel behind their lumbar spine to help reinforce the curve while they are sitting.

My favorite chair is a big ball, the kind now commonly used for exercise. Unlike a conventional chair, the ball always moves a little. It is easier to maintain good alignment when you are moving than when you are static, because your muscles and your brain need to be more awake.

EXERCISE 23: SEATED PSOAS MUSCLE ISOLATION

Prerequisites

Explorations 1 (see page 9), 2 (see page 29), 3 (see page 51), and 6 (see page 135)

Objective

This exercise will give you greater awareness of how your lumbar curve is stabilized by the action of the psoas muscles.

Position

- Sit on a chair (without leaning against the back support), with your legs parallel, and your knees bent at 90 degrees. Place your heals on the ground and the front half of your feet on a phone book, about 2 inches high. Your hands should rest on your thighs. Your weight should be directly over your sit bones, so that your pelvis is level and your lower back is straight.

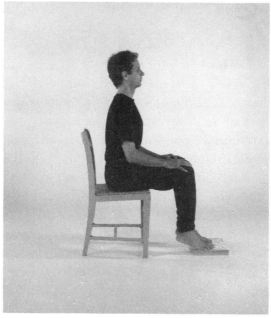

13.1

- As you inhale, slowly raise both heels 2 inches off the floor and keep them up for the duration of the inhalation. As you are raising your heels (and knees), do not press the front of your feet into the phone book. Relax your leg muscles as much as possible. The control of this movement is from the psoas muscle. Ideally, you should feel that your heels and knees are being lifted by the muscles in the front of your hips and lower abdomen, rather than by your thigh or calf muscles. If your psoas muscle is being activated properly, you will feel your pelvis rock forward slightly as your heels lift. This will increase the curve of your lower back slightly.

- As you exhale, slowly return your heels to the floor; press them lightly into the floor for the duration of the exhalation. *Maintain the same long arc in your lower back as when your heels were lifting.*

- Repeat slowly raising and lowering your heels 20 times.

Sensing

Notice how your lumbar curve is increased by the action of the psoas muscles raising the legs slightly. This psoas action is an exaggeration of the ideal muscle use needed to sit properly. When you finish this exercise, notice how you are sitting. Keep the same muscles activated even when your feet rest on the floor. Feel how you can relax your back and entire upper body yet remain nicely upright. This is because your pelvis and lumbar spine are stabilized by your psoas muscles. There is no need to force your shoulders back. This is the secret to comfortable sitting.

Imagining

Imagine that your sit bones are rooted in the chair throughout the exercise.

Walking

Natural walking involves using many of the movements from the exercises in this book. It also involves letting your momentum carry you forward.

When you walk, let your ankles relax. This will encourage your psoas muscles to lift your legs and keep your lower back long at the same time. The psoas are the most important muscles in walking.

Keep your lower back relaxed. Many people habitually tighten their back muscles while walking.

The job of your hip muscles is to allow you to balance on one leg at a time as you walk. With each step, the hip muscles need to relax so that your hips can do their job as shock absorbers and minimize the impact of walking on your upper body. The following exercise will help to strengthen and relax your hips.

Your upper body rotates slightly left and right as you walk. This rotation is carried out primarily by the oblique abdominal muscles (see exploration 5 on page 106).

Keep your shoulders relaxed as you walk. Let your arms swing freely, with as little effort as possible. Also, let the back of your neck relax so your head can move freely. Imagine that your eyes are soft and taking in the world around you.

EXERCISE 24: HIP HIKER

Prerequisite

Exploration 4 (see page 73)

Objective

This exercise both isolates and releases the muscles needed for smooth hip motion when walking.

Position

- Stand with your left leg on a phone book, about 3 inches high. Keep your right leg straight and your right foot hanging next to the book. Place one hand on a wall so you can keep your balance.
- Push your left foot into the book. When you do this, the right side of your pelvis will lift, raising your right leg farther off the ground. Notice how this is done by engaging muscles in the back of your left hip.
- Stop pressing your left foot into the phone book by completely relaxing the left hip muscles you were just using. Your right hip will now drop lower than your left. Lower your right foot until it is flat on the floor, or as close to the floor as possible. Keep both knees straight but not hyperextended. Keep your lower back long.
- Slowly repeat this movement 10 times. Then stand with your right foot on the phone book and repeat 10 more times.

Sensing

Feel the muscles working in the back of your hip, causing the opposite hip to raise and lower. Take a walk around the room, and feel how your hips swing a little to the side when your weight lands on each leg, because your hip muscles are now relaxed.

Imagining

As you are walking, imagine that your leg bones are doing the work, rather than your leg muscles. Let your bones hold you up.

Acknowledgments

THIS BOOK would not have made it beyond the drawing board were it not for the encouragement, coaching, and clear vision of Jonathan Weinert, who took time from his poetry to help me with all things word-related. Ten thousand thanks to you, my friend.

Special thanks to my editor, Beth Frankl, for believing in this book and making it happen.

Thanks to Judy Carl-Hendrick for appearing at just the right time to steer me back on course. My appreciation also goes to Matt Jones, Zev Eisenberg, and Adrian Williamson for help with the photos.

Thank you, Georgia, for your years of encouraging me to do this type of work. Thanks to Nicolas and Adrian for giving their dad the space to write this book.

To all of the friends, family, teachers, clients, and students who have helped me every step of the way, thank you.

I am indebted to the Trust in Diversity Exchange (TIDE) for providing the grant that allowed this project to get underway.

Appendix: Pain Areas

The chart on the following page shows the exercises that are designed to relieve various pain problems. The numbers across the top of the chart refer to the numbered exercises in the book. Locate your pain problem in the left-hand column and you will find marked boxes under the relevant exercises. Remember to do the explorations that are related to each exercise.

EXERCISES TO RELIEVE PAIN

PAIN AREA	1	2	3	4	5	6	7	8	9	10	11	12	13	14	15	16	17	18	19	20	21	22	23	24
Between shoulder blades							✓	✓								✓	✓	✓	✓	✓	✓	✓	✓	✓
Carpal tunnel syndrome														✓	✓	✓	✓	✓	✓					
Fibromyalgia	✓			✓			✓								✓	✓				✓	✓	✓	✓	
Hip pain/bursitis	✓	✓		✓		✓	✓			✓	✓	✓	✓										✓	✓
Knee tendonitis/pain				✓		✓				✓	✓	✓												
Low back pain/arthritis	✓		✓	✓	✓	✓	✓	✓	✓	✓	✓	✓										✓		
Lower neck/upper shoulder pain													✓	✓	✓	✓	✓	✓	✓			✓		
Lumbar disc (bulging)	✓		✓	✓	✓	✓			✓			✓							✓				✓	✓
Muscular groin pain	✓					✓			✓	✓	✓													
Neck pain						✓	✓	✓					✓	✓	✓	✓		✓	✓					
Plantar fascia (foot) pain				✓		✓				✓	✓	✓	✓							✓	✓		✓	✓
Sacroiliac pain		✓		✓		✓			✓	✓	✓	✓	✓							✓				✓
Sciatica	✓	✓	✓	✓	✓	✓			✓	✓		✓	✓							✓				
Shoulder tendonitis/bursitis							✓							✓	✓	✓	✓	✓	✓		✓			
Tension headaches						✓								✓	✓	✓	✓	✓	✓			✓		
Wrist and elbow tendonitis														✓	✓	✓	✓	✓	✓					

Index